WEIGHT LOSS HYPNOSIS FOR WOMEN

WEIGHT LOSS MOTIVATION FOR WOMEN. THE ULTIMATE SUCCESSFUL GUIDE TO GET SLIMMER AND STOP EMOTIONAL EATING.

Fat Burning Happiness

Table of Contents

Introduction

Throughout the world, many people are not comfortable with their weight because of various reasons. Whatever the idea that you have for not being happy with your weight, you must start taking the first step towards a healthy body weight. In this book, you will find many useful tips to help you succeed on your journey to maintaining the right body weight, but there is something that must be stressed. You need to be sure that the kind of weight you desire is according to your body and not looking at the many influencers in the market today. For example, many people around the world struggle to reduce their weight because they want to be like a model they admire on televisions. Others do not even have weight problems, but they end up doing many crazy things to reduce weight because the concept they have about an ideal weight for an individual is wrong. The truth is that different people have different requirements when it comes to their weight and diet. You must be sure that the kind of weight you desire can be achieved depending on your body and it is realistic.

When you have understood yourself, and you know that you have a severe bodyweight problem, you can now follow the steps that are outlined in this book so that you can get the real help that you have been looking for. Many people who desire to reduce their weight would be surprised to find that they are even okay with the weight they have at the moment if they visit a qualified physician. To not be caught in a wave of weight reduction that has no meaning and is propagated by the mainstream media through various advertising agencies. If you fall into this trap, you should know that the frustrations of weight will continue, and you may never find any help because your body is okay. You already understand that there is no ideal weight for all people, but different people have different weights. After evaluating yourself, do you think that you have issues with your weight? Do you feel that you have accumulated excess weight probably due to the bad eating habits that you developed from your childhood? Do you think that it is time for a change, and this change should happen right now? If you feel this way, then you should relax because there is good news.

You may have struggled with the issue of your weight for many years and not found any solution for the problem that you have, but do not worry because this book has all the information that you need when it comes to solving your weight problems. You need to understand that the change you are looking for may not happen immediately because it is something that takes time, and it requires patience and dedication. Those who have succeeded in the past following the guided meditation methods can attest to the fact that this change, growth, and development need the necessary work. Before you can dive to studying and mastering the meditation techniques listed in this book, you must be prepared to maintain your discipline and promise yourself that you will not break them. Always ensure you are strict with the meditations that you decide to include in your weight loss program because it is the best way to ensure that you achieve the results that you desire. Throughout this book, you will find that discipline is being emphasized, and this is deliberate since it will help you greatly in sticking to what you have chosen, and eventually, you will start seeing the results.

Many people who have found them useful have practised the meditation exercises found in this book, and you should hope that they would benefit you. If others have used them and succeeded in their journey to lose weight, then it means that if you are focused, and you keep your concentration. When you do these meditations properly, you will be able to connect your body and mind and find that you experience a feeling of calmness. You have the will power to achieve not only your weight goal but also the various aspects of your life. This book is helpful to you in many ways because you will not only find success in weight reduction but also you will experience better holistic health.

Chapter 1

Love Your Body and Your Soul

Glad individuals acknowledge and love themselves regardless of what their body resembles, irrespective of how they feel. An ideal organization isn't preferred or all the more empowering over a body not considered immaculate by the "powers that be." Your magnificence originates from inside.

Consider somebody you know (or knew) who isn't generally all that appealing; however, who appears to adore herself so much that she feels delightful and acts as needs be. Individuals like that tend to be well known. Curiously, their excellence sparkles so splendidly that they seem, by all accounts, to be alluring to others.

Individuals in the media don't typically seem as though they seem to look in front of an audience or magazines and films. That is the reason the calling of make-up specialists exists. In my mind, what they do is make-up how this individual will appear to the crowd and fans. When photograph distributing is included, nobody is viewed as they look. All pictures get finished up.

At the point when you love yourself, honestly and genuinely love yourself, regardless of how old you develop to be your sentiments about you won't change. The fascinating piece about adoring yourself is living in a condition of satisfaction. Hardly any individuals get the chance to abide there—the individuals who do remain youthful until the end of time.

Tips To Assist You with Adoring Your Body

1. Take power back to characterize your Beauty-

You are not just taking it back for the social/media definitions yet in addition to individuals around you in your life who have offered critical comments about your body. These individuals couldn't see the magnificence of your body since they had retained the standard definitions themselves-and were deciding for you and most likely their body against these gauges too. Pause for a minute presently to close your eyes and envision reclaiming the power to characterize the excellence of your body. Take it once again from the social definitions and the media-in your mental state, "I won't permit you to characterize what my body ought to resemble any longer." Think back to individuals that had offered negative remarks to you about your body-a relative, a sentimental accomplice, or different children when you were close to nothing. State to them in your mind, "I reclaim the power to characterize the magnificence of my body-your remarks were bends and false, and I no longer give them any power." Feel how great this feels to free yourself from the entirety of this cynicism.

2. Clear Your Negative Beliefs about Your Body-

Due to your introduction to the social molding about the alleged perfect female body-you presumably have rehearsed self-judgment of your body for not fitting in with the advanced "perfect." These decisions and negative convictions are again contortions and not founded on the reality of the one of your very kind stunner body. We, as a whole, have groups of various sizes and shapes that are uncommon and genuinely delightful.

Relinquish your unbending convictions about how your body should look and start to perceive how the very things that are diverse about your body are the very things that make you one of a kind and lovely. Record the negative messages that you state to yourself about your body. Envision thinking of them to discharge them from your cognizance. Get them hard and fast the most negative terrible ones you can consider. Take a gander at these messages-notice how you could never fantasy about directing these sentiments toward any other person in your life. Take a gander at all of these messages and apologize to your body, saying, "I'm sorry to such an extent that I directed these harmful sentiments toward you-I guarantee that I won't direct these sentiments toward you again and I will begin adoring you." Look at these messages again and with an expectation to completely discharge them-destroy the piece of paper and discard it. A few people like to fabricate a fire outside and consume the document as a method of releasing this cynicism.

3. Exercise for the Joy of Feeling Your Body Move-

At the point when you exercise to take out fat from your body as well as to make up for calories, eaten-this can emerge out of a position of fear and have a vitality of attempting to control and battle against your body. Envision practicing for the delight of moving your body and from a goal to be wanting to your body-a craving for it to be sound and have more vitality. The customers I work with around this issue will, in general, have the option to keep up an activity program if they do it from a position of satisfaction and self-love as opposed to control and fear about their weight.

Notice if there are things throughout your life that you don't accomplish for fear of individuals seeing your body-like swimming, moving, or some other movement. Remind yourself that you have the right to do the things you appreciate regardless of your shape. Relinquish what others consider you and remain concentrated on the way that you reserve each option to do the things you understand.

4. Remind Yourself What the Purpose of Having a Body Is-

Your body is yours to encounter life; ultimately, to take it in and appreciate it. Your body is a vehicle for you to encounter existence with the entirety of your faculties. Your body permits you: to feel a warm breeze on your skin, feel the cold water in a lake when you swim, see the entirety of the striking shades of nightfall, hear the whole of the excellence of the music, to listen to the hints of fowls and trees moving in the breeze, feel the non-abrasiveness of somebody's hand, feel the delight of moving, taste and appreciate flavorful food, communicate through a grin, tears or giggling. Your body is for you, for nobody else to investigate or pass judgment. You are not here as a presentation for other people; however, as a wholly encapsulated person with more profound, more extravagant characteristics than merely your appearance.

5. at the point when you look in The Mirror-Look at Yourself through Loving Eyes-

For some, ladies glancing in the mirror transforms into an activity of self-judgment. They focus on the entirety of their apparent flaws and what they feel is "off-base" with their body or face. Again the models they are deciding for themselves against is this ridiculous perfect that is advanced in the media. I have numerous customers who, when they previously began working with me, said that they couldn't glance in the mirror since all they saw were these apparent flaws. I recommend that they move this by instead taking a gander at themselves in the mirror through adoring eyes. A model would be if you look in the mirror and see a wrinkle that you would generally judge-see this wrinkle with affection and empathy - and even observe the excellence of this wrinkle. Set an away from to see yourself through the perspective of adoration - intrude on the self-judgment and move into being exceptionally cherishing with yourself. This will be something that you have to rehearse before it turns into a propensity. Yet, it will be justified even despite the exertion since you will start to feel extremely magnificent about yourself.

6. Have Your Self-Esteem be Internally Referenced

Have your self-regard be founded on your interior characteristics as opposed to your outside appearance. What are the features that make you-you? Is it your sympathy, your new innovativeness, your insight, your ability to have a ton of fun, your awareness, your perceptiveness, your ability to tune in to individuals, or your caring heart? Think about the individuals that you love in your life. You love them for what their identity is - the one of a kind Spirit that they are - not for what they resemble. That is how they feel about you-they love you for what your identity is and the entirety of the extraordinary characteristics that make up you. Figure out how to esteem yourself for the substance of you - not for the physical structure that you travel around in.

7. Investigate the deeper purpose behind the distraction with your appearance/weight.

Here and there, when somebody is engrossed with their appearance, it might be a shirking system for more profound, increasingly agonizing sentiments. Check-in with yourself and check whether this may be the situation. If in your youth things were excruciating for you and crazy, you may have figured out how to concentrate on your weight as an approach to keep away from the forlornness and defenselessness of what was going on around you. Or then again, perhaps there is a problematic issue in your life today that you don't have the fearlessness to confront like a problematic relationship or absence of direction in your life. A distraction with your appearance occupies you from facing these issues. If so, for you, it is significant for you to get support for yourself to open up to confront these sentiments straightforwardly. You can get this help through facing the challenge to uncover your feelings to a confided in companion or working with an advocate who can assist you with working through these emotions.

8. Take out Comparing Yourself to Others-

The vitality of correlation and rivalry is damaging to yourself and the other individual. Doing this is simply one more type of putting yourself and won't help you to feel better; however, it will exacerbate you think even. Pledge to pass on this sort of vitality. Instead, if you see somebody who is appealing as opposed to contrasting yourself with this individual or making a decision about them-state instead, "She is alluring as am I." Celebrate that other individual and yourself as well. You will discover this feels such a significant amount of superior to contrasting yourself with them or being basic.

9. Take One of the Areas of Your Body You Typically Judge and Take a Week to Fully Love This Part of You

Go through 15 minutes daily taking a gander at this piece of your body, and discover things to adore about it, even better, do it for the day. The additionally testing it is to do this, the more you have to do it! I read in a book about a lady who did this activity, and following seven days of doing it, an outsider came up to her and revealed to her how delightful this piece of her body was! At the point when we change our particular manner of seeing ourselves - it changes the style in which others see us also. You need your first expectation of doing this activity to be simply the move in your affection, not to have an impact on how others see you. How you see you are continually going to be what is generally significant.

10. Conclude That You Are Beautiful and Practice Being Beautiful

You get the chance to choose if you are lovely or not. If, as I expressed above, you have returned your power to characterize yourself, then why not guarantee your magnificence! Take a day and rehash to yourself, "I am Beautiful." Do things that cause you to feel excellent, wear something exceptional that you love, and feel extraordinary in. Walk like you are lovely. Glance in the mirror and state, "I am excellent." This may feel unbalanced from the start yet keep on doing this until you truly begin to trust it. Commend what your identity is and your beautiful, exceptional body. We need ladies who are seeing and praising their excellence; it helps other ladies who are stuck in pessimism about their body see that there is another increasingly euphoric way to take - the idea of genuine self-love!

Chapter 2
How Does the Mind Work

Your mind plays a critical role in helping you get healthy, get in shape, and stay that way. Your account is so vital that if you can't get your mind to cooperate with your body, you could be seriously undermining your chances at improving your overall health and wellbeing.

Often getting your head in line with your body is dependent on being able to make the most of your internal programming mechanism. In other words, what you tell yourself is vital to achieving anything you want. This self-talk can make, or break, your chances at becoming who you want to be.

For example, if you are continually telling yourself that you are not up to the task, that you are never going to make it, or that it is simply too hard to, then the chances of you not achieving your goals will be very slim. In contrast, if your self-talk is based upon your understanding of what it takes to be the best version of yourself, then the chances of you achieving anything that you want can explode through the roof. Best of all, you will give yourself a fighting chance when it comes to warding off any unwanted thoughts and feelings.

Also, it is vital to consider the fact that input from external sources can wreak havoc on your self-confidence and the way your mind process such data. You might get negative messages from people around you, or even attacks upon your choice of a healthy lifestyle. In some cases, attacks go to such extremes that some people stop talking to you, or decide not to hang out with you anymore, simply because you don't partake in eating or drinking binges.

These are people that you don't need in your life. It is best to surround yourself with like-minded people who will support you and help you in your endeavors. In doing so, you will be able to make better choices and stay on track.

Ultimately, you have the power to get on track and stay there. You don't need to depend on anything to help you make the most of your abilities to get in shape, drop some pounds and improve your overall health and wellbeing. Sure, it helps to be surrounded by supportive friends and family. But in the end, you have everything you need to be successful.

Throughout this book, we are going to be looking at how you can summon that inner willpower that you have to aid you in making the most of any changes that you need to make… and help them stick. After all, anyone can go on one of those crash diets. But what will help you truly become what you want to be is your desire and willingness to make things happen. That, coupled with a robust methodology, such as the power of meditation, you will come to develop your winning formula. You can think that this isn't a cookie-cutter solution. This is the type of approach which you can build for yourself. That means that what you do, what you choose to accomplish, and the way that you decide to do it will be your own, particular way of doing things. That will surely guarantee that what you do will be both successful and sustainable.

With that in your back pocket, you can feel confident about moving on to bigger and better things in your life. You won't have to worry about being successful ever again simply because you have already achieved the most critical goal in your life. Based on that, you can begin to feel comfortable in your skin. And there is nothing better than feeling good about yourself while making the best of your opportunity to achieve everything that you have always wanted to achieve.

Chapter 3
Why is it hard to Lose Weight

For anyone who has ever struggled with weight, life can seem like an uphill battle. It can be downright devastating to see how difficult it can be to turn things around and shed some weight.

The fact of the matter is that losing weight doesn't have to be an uphill battle. Most of this requires you to understand better why this struggle happens and what you can do to help give yourself a fighting chance.

Physiological factors are affecting your ability to lose weight. There are also psychological, emotional and even spiritual causes that affect your overall body's ability to help you lose weight and reach your ideal weight levels.

The Obvious Culprits

The obvious culprits that are holding you back are diet, a lack of exercise and a combination of both.

First off, your diet plays a crucial role in your overall health and wellbeing. When it comes to weight management, your diet has everything to do with your ability to stay in shape and ward of unwanted weight.

When it comes to diet, we are not talking about keto, vegan, or Atkins; we are talking about the common foods which you consume and the amounts that you have of each one which is why diet is one of the obvious culprits. If you have a diet that is high in fat, high in sodium and high in sugar, you can rest assured that your body will end up gaining weight at a rapid rate.

When you consume high amounts of sugar, carbs and fats, your body transforms them into glucose which storing it in the body as fat. Of course, a proportion of the glucose produced by your body is used up as energy. However, if you consume far more than you need, your body isn't going to get rid of it; your body is going to hold on to it and make sure that it is stored for a rainy day.

Here is another vital aspect to consider: sweet and salty foods, the kind that we love so dearly, trigger "happy hormones" in the brain, namely dopamine. Dopamine is a hormone that is released by the body when it "feels good". And food is one of the best ways to trigger it, which is why you somehow feel better after eating your favorite meals. It also explains the reason why we resort to food when we are not feeling well which is called "comfort food", and it is one of the most popular coping mechanisms employed by folks around the world.

This rush of dopamine causes a person to become addicted to food. As with any addiction, there comes a time when you need to get more and more of that same substances to meet your body's requirements.

As a result of diet, a lack of regular exercise can do a number on your ability to lose weight and maintain a healthy balance. What regular exercise does is increase your body's overall caloric requirement. As such, your metabolism needs to convert fat at higher rates to keep up with your body's energy demands.

As the body's energetic requirements increase, that is, as your exercise regimen gets more and more intense, you will find that you will need increased amounts of both oxygen and glucose which is one of the reasons why you feel hungrier when you ramp up your workouts.

However, increased caloric intake isn't just about consuming more and more calories for the sake of consuming more and more calories; you need to consume an equal amount of proteins, carbs, fats and vitamins too for your body to build the necessary elements that will build muscle, foster movement and provide proper oxygenation in the blood.

Moreover, nutrients are required for the body to recover. One of the byproducts of exercise is called "lactic acid". Lactic acid builds up in the muscles as they get more and more tired. Lactic acid signals the body that it is time to stop working out or risk injury if you continue. Without lactic acid, your body would have no way of knowing when your muscles have overextended their capacity.

After you have completed your workout, the body needs to get rid of the lactic acid buildup. So, if you don't have enough of the right minerals in your body, for example, potassium, your muscles will ache for days until your body is finally able to get rid of the lactic acid buildup. This example goes to show how proper nutrition is needed to help the body get moving and also recover once it is done exercising.

As a result, a lack of exercise reconfigures your body's metabolism to work at a slower pace. What that means is that you need to consume fewer calories to fuel your body's lack of exercise. So, if you end up wasting more than you need, your body will just put it away for a rainy day. Plain and simple.

The Sneaky Culprits

The sneaky culprits are the ones that aren't quite so overt in causing you to gain weight or have trouble shedding pounds. These culprits hide beneath the surface but are very useful when it comes to keeping you overweight. The first culprit we are going to be looking at is called "stress".

Stress is a potent force. From an evolutionary perspective, it exists as a means of fueling the flight-or-fight response. Stress is the human response to danger. When a person senses danger, the body begins to secrete a hormone called "cortisol". When cortisol begins running through the body, it signals the entire system to prep for a potential showdown. Depending on the situation, it might be best to hightail it out and live to fight another day.

In our modern way of life, stress isn't so much a response to life and death situations (though it can certainly be). Instead, it is the response to cases that are deemed as "conflictive" by the mind. This could be a confrontation with a co-worker, bumper to bumper traffic, or any other type of situation in which a person feels vulnerable in some way.

Throughout our lives, we subject to countless interactions in which we must deal with stress. In general terms, the feelings of alertness subside when the perceived threat is gone. However, when a person is exposed to prolonged periods of stress, any number of changes can happen.

One such change is overexposure to cortisol. When there is too much cortisol in the body, the body's overall response is to hoard calories, increase the production of other hormones such as adrenaline and kick up the immune system's function.

This response by the body is akin to the panic response that the body would assume when faced with prolonged periods of hunger or fasting. As a result, the body needs to go into survival mode. Please bear in mind that the body has no clue if it is being chased by a bear, dealing with a natural disaster or just having a bad day at the office. Regardless of the circumstances, the body is faced with the need to ensure its survival. So, anything that it eats goes straight to fat stores.

Moreover, a person's stressful situation makes them search for comfort and solace. There are various means of achieving this. Food is one of them. So is alcohol consumption. These two types of pleasures lead to significant use of calories. Again, when the body is in high gear, it will store as many calories and keep them in reserve.

This what makes you gain weight when you are stressed out.

Another of the sneaky culprits is sleep deprivation. In short, sleep deprivation is sleeping less than the recommended 8 hours that all adults should sleep. In the case of children, the recommended amount of sleep can be anywhere from 8 to 12 hours, depending on their age.

Granted, some adults can function perfectly well with less than 8 hours' sleep. Some folks can work perfectly well with 6 hours' sleep while there are folks who are shattered when they don't get eight or even more hours' sleep. This is different for everyone as each individual is different in this regard.

That being said, sleep deprivation can trigger massive amounts of cortisol. This, fueled by ongoing exposure to stress, leads the body to further deepening its panic mode. When this occurs, you can rest assured that striking a healthy balance between emotional wellbeing and physical health can be nearly impossible to achieve.

Now, the best way to overcome sleep deprivation is to get sleep. But that is easier said than done. One of the best ways to get back on track to a certain degree is to get in enough sleep when you can.

The last sneaky culprit on our list is emotional distress. Emotional distress can occur as a result of any number of factors. For example, the loss of a loved one, a stressful move, a divorce, or the loss of a job can all contribute to large amounts of emotional distress. While all of the situations mentioned above begin as a stressful situation, they can fester and lead to severe psychological issues. Over time, these emotional issues can grow into more profound topics such as General Anxiety Disorder or Depression. Studies have shown that prolonged periods of stress can lead to depression and a condition known as Major Depression.

The most common course of treatment for anxiety and depression is the use of an antidepressant. And, guess what: one of the side effects associated with antidepressants is the weight. The reason for this is that antidepressant tinker with the brain's chemistry in such a way that they alter the brains processing of chemicals through the suppression of serotonin transport. This causes the brain to readjust its overall chemistry. Thus, you might find the body unable to process food quite the same way. In general, it is common to see folks gain as much as 10 pounds as a result of taking antidepressants.

As you can see, weight gain is not the result of "laziness" or being "undisciplined". Sure, you might have to clean up your diet somewhat and get more exercise. But the causes we have outlined here ought to provide you with enough material to see why there are less obvious causes that are keeping yours from achieving your ideal weight. This is why meditation plays such a key role in helping you deal with stress and emotional strife while helping you find a balance between your overall mental and physical wellbeing.

Ultimately, the strategies and techniques that we will further outline in this book will provide you with the tools that will help you strike that balance and eventually lead you to find the most effective way in which you will deal with the rigors of your day to day life while being able to make the most out of your efforts to lead a healthier life. You have everything you need to do it. So, let's find out how you can achieve this.

Chapter 4
The Importance of Genetics

How You Were Raised, Counts

Those who have been overweight all their lives go through individual cycles. There is a period of unhealthy habits, the recognition that there needs to be a change, an attempt at reform, the failure to follow through, and then back to a period of unhealthy habits. This cycle is present in many people that are overweight, but for those that were overweight kids and teens, it might be better understood. We might have also adopted this unhealthy cycle from our parents. Once we've found ourselves in this dangerous position, it can feel like clawing our way out when we decide we want to lose weight. If the pattern of behavior is not at first recognized, then we won't be able to determine the best method of breaking this unhealthy habit.

Studies have proven that kids who were weight-shamed go through cycles of binge eating and meal skipping that leads to self-loathing. A child that experiences criticism from their parents will start learning unhealthy methods of coping with weight and dieting. Eating is something that we've been doing all our lives, so the way that we eat now is undoubtedly related to the way that we used to be taught to eat. Parents that might have body-shamed their kids by telling them they needed to lose weight or stop eating so much are responsible for causing self-loathing later in life.

Weight-shaming is not just blatantly telling someone that they are fat. It might also cloud diet encouragement. If your mom or dad always told you to try out a diet or suggested that you shouldn't eat a particular food, which was probably enough for you to feel a certain amount of shame about your weight. Even having a parent that continually talks about dieting is likely to make a child feel as though they should diet, too.

Many kids might grow up with moms who are always trying out new diets and fads. By seeing this is a kid, we end up going through the same phases. Maybe a parent was always saying things like, "I need to start my diet on Monday." This idea gets it in the kid's head that diets are something they should aim for, but only at a moment of convenience. The way a parent or even older sibling always talked about their body will play into how you might see your own body now. Perhaps your mom was still saying things like, "I hate my thighs; they are so big!" If a girl looks in the mirror and sees she has the same- shaped thighs as her mother, she'll end up thinking about how both she and her mother see those thighs as significant, even though the mother never said anything directly to the girl about her body.

It is challenging because most parents think they are helping. Parents that stock the fridge with Diet Coke instead of regular might think they are doing everyone a favor when really, they are still supplying a form of addiction. Those that make sure to weigh their kids or track their workout routines could be doing so just because they want to make sure their kid is healthy. Still, they might not realize they are setting them up in a fearful manner in which dieting and exercising are an authoritative issue. Parents who are strict with routines might raise kids that don't have any method at all as an act of rebellion.

How our parents diet, exercise, and talk about health, in general, will also form our body perceptions. A daughter of a mother who consistently crashes diets and works out too hard will likely produce a daughter that does the same. A father that only eats microwave meals or fast food is setting his kids up for doing the same when they become adults. When this happens, it is an insidious issue that we might not even recognize. The things our parents do can seem reasonable to us, as it is behavior that we learn is standard.

Be mindful of how you talk about exercise around children. Whether they are your kids or someone else's, never talk about body issues around kids. If you walk around talking about how much you hate your belly flab, you are teaching the kids around you to evaluate their stomachs, wondering if they, too, have too much belly flab. Kids will be confronted with these body issues in other ways, as it is inevitable. As parents, caretakers, or any role models, we should be teaching our kids how to love their bodies and adequately take care of them because they deserve to be healthy, not because they should be skinnier or prettier.

Pregnant Moms Who Exercise Will Likely Give Birth to Healthy Kids

A study was conducted in which one group of pregnant rats were given exercise wheels, while another group of pregnant rats wasn't assigned anything. Those who used the exercise wheels ended up giving birth to more active babies. The babies of the moms that didn't work out would sit around and not do anything, as opposed to the babies of the moms that were always using an exercise wheel, who would use the wheel themselves. This was true for at least half of the rats born from active mothers. They weren't given anything else, so there weren't any factors to determine the difference in the level of activity other than the environment in which they were raised in the womb.

This exercise was inspired by similar research done on humans, though many scientists wonder if the effects were just because of a mother's influence after birth. Instead of assuming that it was from active pregnancy, many scientists speculate that the difference in the amount of desire for physical activity is because mothers with active pregnancies are also mothers with busy lives. Their lifestyle and habits can affect children, but the study with the rats proves that it might be on a level different than just the learned behavior.

Even in the womb, our mothers are teaching us how to exercise. We learn before we're also walking how vital exercise is in maintaining a high level of physical activity. If a mother is more active while she's pregnant, she's setting her unborn baby up for a future in which it is just generally more productive. This means that not only are we affected by the learned habits of our parents, but how we are actually created and grown also determines how much physical activity we let into our life.

Look back on your mother, father, or any other person that helped raise you, biologically or not. Were they active? Did they let that level of activity negatively affect your life? Did they reject exercise and healthy eating at all costs? Did you learn your unhealthy eating habits, or are they just a product of not being taught anything at all? We are taught how to eat and exercise, which means we are also taught how not to eat healthily or use. We can't entirely blame our parents for the way we live now, but it is still essential to recognize as it'll help bring us closer to closure with the unhealthy person in our head.

This is the right motivation for any woman hoping to get pregnant in the future. Starting a family is a goal for many different people. An essential aspect of starting that family is making sure to have a high level of physical activity. Kids require a lot of chasing and lifting. It is much harder for those that are not in shape to look after and give proper attention to active kids. It is also essential to be healthy when pregnant with them to get them started right away with a healthy lifestyle. After kids are born, parents are also responsible for making sure their kids understand how to live a healthy lifestyle that does not include any bad habits.

Chapter 5
Changing Your Mindset

Why a Rigid and Aggressive Approach Doesn't Work

When it comes to making any sort of the change in life, the approach you take will make or break your success. If you choose a strategy that doesn't work well with your specific personality, the likelihood of relapse occurring will be extremely high. We will discuss the drawbacks of approaching change with an aggressive and rigid approach.

Taking an approach that is focused on perfection leaves you feeling down on yourself and like a failure most of the time. Because this causes you to notice that you are not perfect instead of focusing on the right parts, the progress you have made will always make you feel like you are not doing enough or that you have not made enough progress. Since you will never achieve perfection as this is impossible for anyone, you will never feel satisfaction or allow yourself to celebrate your achievements. You must recognize that this will be something complicated, but that you will do it anyways. If you force yourself into change like a drill sergeant and with an aggressive mindset, you will end up beating yourself up every day for something. Pushing yourself will not lead to a long-lasting change, as you will eventually become fed up with all of the rules you have placed on yourself, and you will just want to abandon the entire mission. If you approach the change with rigidity, you will not allow yourself time to look back on your achievements and celebrate yourself, to have a tasty meal that is good for your soul every once in a while, and you may fall off of your plan in a more extreme way than you were before. You may end up having a week-long binge and dropping down into worse habits than you had back.

Your mindset plays a huge role in your success when it comes to change. The way that you view your journey will make or break it and will determine whether or not your change is lasting or fleeting, and whether or not you become invested in making the changes in your life. While you need to push yourself to do anything hard, the key is knowing when to ease up on yourself a little bit and when to push harder. Recognizing and responding to this is much more useful than putting your nose to the grindstone every day and becoming burnt out, tired, and left without any more willpower. Continuing in this challenging journey that a lifestyle change involves, you must give yourself a break now and then. Think of this like running a marathon, where you will need to go about it slowly and purposefully with a strategy in mind. If you ran into a marathon full-speed and refused to slow down or look back at all, you would lose energy, stamina, and motivation in quite a short amount of time and turn back or run off the side of the road feeling defeated and as if you failed. Looking at this example, you can see that this person did not fail. They just approached the marathon with the wrong strategy and that they would have been completely capable of finishing that marathon if they had taken their time, followed a plan, and slowed down every once in a while to regain their strength. Even if they walked the marathon slowly for hours and hours, eventually, they would make it over that finish line. They would probably also do so feeling proud, accomplished, and like a new person. This is how we want to view this journey or any journey of self-improvement. Even if you take only one tiny step each day, you are making a step toward your goal, and that is the crucial part.

The Deprivation Trap

There is a term when it comes to dieting that is called The Deprivation Trap. The deprivation trap is something that can occur when you approach dieting with a strict mindset. What this means is that you become stuck in a type of thinking trap within your mind. In this type of thinking, you become focused on what you can't have and what you are restricting yourself off. You become hyper-focused on everything you can't allow yourself to have and become resentful of the fact that you aren't able just to eat what you want. After a while, because you are focusing so intently on what you can't have and the fact that you can't have it, you decide that you are just going to have it anyway, or just have a little bit of it, out of a feeling of anger and entitlement. The next thing you know, you have gone on a binge, and after restricting yourself entirely for some time, you have now undone that in a single sitting. You will then begin to feel terrible about yourself and what you have done, and you begin to feel like you need to punish yourself. Thus can start the cycle of deprivation.

Further, it is quite challenging to avoid this when you are trying to make a change by using deprivation. It is quite rare that a person, no matter how strong their willpower, will be able to deprive themselves of something without easing off of it ultimately. A sudden and strict deprivation is not natural to our brains and will leave us feeling confused and frustrated.

How to Overcome the Deprivation Trap

To avoid the deprivation trap, or overcome it if you are already finding yourself there, there are things that we can do and approaches we can take that will set us up better for success.

To avoid this trap, the first thing we must do is prevent complete deprivation of anything. Instead of depriving ourselves of something ultimately, we will instead try to make better choices, one meal or one snack at a time. Focusing on small parts of our day or lower sections of our lives will help us to motivate ourselves. This is because looking forward to the rest of our lives and thinking that we will never be able to have a sure thing again is quite an overwhelming thought, especially if this is something that we enjoy. Therefore, we must instead look at it like "I will make a better choice for my lunch today," and then all you need to focus on is lunch, not the entire rest of your life.

Strategies for the Mind

Like we all know and read in some websites about weight-loss, easing into a lifestyle change is the best way to go about something like this because of the way that our minds work. We don't like looking forward to our lives and feeling like we will have no control over what we are going to do with it. By choosing smaller sections to break it up into, we can be more present in each moment, which makes making healthy choices easier. By doing so, all of these small sections add up to weeks, months, and eventually years of healthy options. Finally, we have gone a year without turning to sweets in a moment of sadness and only chosen them when we are consciously choosing to treat ourselves.

Another strategy that we can use for our minds is to reward yourself at milestones along your journey. At one week you can reward yourself with a date night at a restaurant, or at one month you can visit the new bakery down the street. This not only helps you to stay motivated because you are allowing yourself some of the joys you love, but it also keeps you motivated because you are allowing yourself to take time to look back at how far you have come and feel great about your progress. Allowing yourself to celebrate goes hand in hand with this, as well. When you make the right choice or plan what you will order at a restaurant before you get there, allowing yourself to feel happy and proud is very important. By doing this, you are showing yourself that you have done something great, that you are capable of making changes, and that you will allow yourself to feel good about these positive strides you have made instead of just looking to the next one all the time. If you were to ignore this and be of the mindset that nothing is good enough, you would end up feeling burnt out and entirely down about the length of the process. Think of that marathon analogy again, and this is what can happen if we don't allow ourselves time to feel proud and accomplished for small victories along the way.

Another strategy for the mind is to avoid beating yourself up for falling off the wagon. This may happen sometimes. What we need to do, though, is to focus not on the fact that it has happened, but on how we are going to deal with and react to it. There are a variety of reactions that a person can have to this. We will examine the possible responses and the pros and cons below:

One is that they feel as though their progress is ruined and that they might as well begin another time again, so they go back to their old ways and may not try again for some time. This could happen many times over as they will fall off each time and then decide that they might as well give up this time and try again, but each time it ends the same.

Two, the person could fall off of their diet plan and tell themselves that this day is a write-off and that they will begin the next day again. The problem with this method is that continuing the rest of the day as you would have before you decided to make a change will make it so that the next day is like beginning all over again, and it will be tough to start again. They may be able to start the next day again, and it could be fine, but they must be able to motivate themselves if they are to do this. Knowing that you have fallen off makes it so that you may feel down on yourself and feel as though you can't do it, so beginning again the next day is significant.

And they then decide that they will pick it up again the next week. This will be even harder than starting the next day again as multiple days of eating whatever you like will make it very hard to go back to making the healthy choices still afterwards.

Four, after eating something that they wish they hadn't, and that wasn't a healthy choice, they will decide not to eat anything for the rest of the day so that they don't eat too many calories or too much sugar, and decide that the next day they will begin again. This is very difficult on the body as you are going to be quite hungry by the time bed rolls around. Instead of forgiving yourself, you are punishing yourself, and it will make it very hard not to reach for chips late at night when you are starving and feeling down.

Number five is what you should do in this situation. This option is the best for success and will make it the most likely that you will succeed long-term. The key to staying on track can bounce back. The people who can bounce back mentally are the ones who will be most likely to succeed. You will need to maintain a positive mental state and look forward to the rest of the day and the rest of the week in just the same way as you did before you had a slip-up.

Chapter 6
Overcome Your Weight Loss Plateau

There's no room for error when you set yourself up with strict, black and white guidelines to abstain entirely from those foods. You are on or off the diet, either. You're off the wagon once you've had the cookie—and that means anything goes. What's the difference between two and twelve cookies? Next week you will continue the sugar ban again — or probably next month.

Here's the worst part: the guilt, embarrassment, and self-criticism resulting from "breaking the rules" that prevent you from making reasonable efforts. It may sound like self-sabotage, but it's very logical in fact: if you realize you're punishing yourself for failure, why try? Who needs punishment? In our curriculum, we refer to ourselves as the Inner Critic, the self-critical element. It's a cruel inner voice that focuses on only one part of ourselves—such as a sugar weakness—with a meanness heart, without looking at the bigger picture of who we are. The criticism of getting dishes from the Inner Critic causes one to feel worse and have less desire to adjust. If it's so frustrating to our accumulated experience trying to improve our actions, we stop working. Health psychologists refer to the "abstinence violation effect" spiral of failure-shame-avoidance, which results from violating rigid rules.

Health Happens "In the Middle"

It's unusual that our days go exactly as expected – at work, at home, and anywhere in between. Our children get sick; we get sick; we get stuck in the traffic; we get bad news about the wellbeing of a friend; our supervisor adds a job to our overflowing plate.

Not only is the diet mentality detrimental to weight loss and physical wellbeing; it also runs counter to emotional health. The word cognitive rigidity is used by psychologists to describe thought patterns which are so entrenched that people have difficulty thinking flexibly. Humans are not robots. It's natural to have a hard time implementing a strict plan — whether it's a diet, a "detox," or an effort to give up sugar in cold-turkey. In an ever-changing environment, versatility is key to maintaining healthy eating habits.

The entire notion of versatility is frightening for many people who have struggled with their eating habits, bringing to mind an "everything goes" mindset that can do nothing but curb their unhealthy habits. And that preoccupation is correct. We don't say "anything goes." Having plenty of freedom but no expectations or guidance can leave us wandering in our attempts to make changes — we don't even know where to begin. How then, without being locked into a fixed program, can you make changes?

Behavior-changing progress is most successful when individuals are "in the middle" and not at the extremes. It is crucial to have goals and expectations. However, there is still enough flexibility to allow you to adjust to changing circumstances — including getting off track — to improve your eating habits and continue those changes. It runs counter to the mindset of the diet, and contrary to "everything goes "—and is sustainable.

Get Moving Mindfully

Like healthy food, physical activity (and its lack) plays a significant role in our general wellbeing, our risk of illness, our mental health and happiness, and our weight, of course. But as with food, trends are troubling over the last fifty years, with more and more people living sedentary lives. The numbers are different, but they're grim. Surveys show that just 20 per cent of American adults say they follow the fitness requirements for exercise and strength training, according to the Centers for Disease Control, but the truth could be much worse. Researchers at the National Cancer Institute, who used motion sensors to monitor people more accurately, found that only 5% had at least 30 minutes of moderate-intensity exercise most days of the week.

In January, new participants who plan to work out are filling the gym every day. In the short term, this method can be very motivating but is generally not sustainable. Once again, it's the power-through-it approach, based on external motivation and punishment/reward (think of "no pain, no benefit" and the glistening, unattainable bodies on show in running-shoe ads). To others, starting is too daunting, while many others start and then fizzle out. And some people are overdoing exercise, which can be as harmful as underdoing it. Both of these trends are indicators of shifting outward-in approach.

There is a safe, middle way that begins with yourself tuning in. The why of exercise, as with food, tells them how. Tell yourself, "What motivates me to exercise? Who do I do this for? "May provide significant detail. For example, you might realize you've been jogging to keep up with (and maybe impress) your athletic sister-in-law, but you don't enjoy it—and what you love is dancing. What if you viewed physical activity as an opportunity to help your overall wellbeing? What if you gain strength, bring joy and fun, and feel confident and competent, instead of concentrating on a specific target (losing a certain amount of weight or fitting into a certain dress), or seeing exercise as something you "should" do? What if you just did it for yourself?

Instead of concentrating on the result, you should focus on the process—miles jogged, pounds lost, calories burned. That means adapting to the way your body feels before, during, and after exercise. That lets you stay versatile. If you know that when swimming your shoulder gets stiff, you should stop before it is an injury — and maybe change your routine to include other activities as well. It helps to differ between a few events for most people, both to avoid damage and to keep off boredom. If you're feeling resistant to the thought of exercise, consider why you're exercising—what you want in the long run. Rather than telling yourself, "Do I feel like doing some exercise?" Mind why this is important to you.

When done in a safe, conscientious way, exercise for a simple purpose is a positive feedback loop: it feels fantastic! And though when you're exercising you feel any pain or exhaustion, you'll experience the benefits shortly after. In fact, with exercise, sometimes the effects are felt faster than with changes in the diet. Our bodies and brains—all from our blood vessels and mitochondria to the feel-good neurotransmitters in our mind—function better when we frequently travel about. It's vital for self-care and overall wellbeing to find your way to the right routine — not too little, not too much, and something you enjoy.

Chapter 7
What is Self-Hypnosis?

If you can afford to undergo a series of hypnotherapy session with a specialist, you may do so. This is ideal as you will work with a professional who can guide you through the treatment and will also provide you with valuable advice on nutrition and exercises.

Clinical Hypnotherapy

When first meeting with a therapist, they start by explaining you the type of hypnotherapy he or she is using. Then you will discuss your personal goals so the therapist can better understand your motivations.

The formal session will start with your therapist, speaking in a gentle and soothing voice. This will help you relax and feel safe during the entire therapy. Once your mind is more receptive, the therapist will start suggesting ways that can help you modify your exercise or eating habits as well as other ways to help you reach your weight loss goals.

Specific words or repetition of particular phrases can help you at this stage. The therapist may also help you in visualizing the body image you want, which is one effective technique in hypnotherapy.

To end the session, the therapist will bring you out from the hypnotic stage, and you will start to be more alert. Your personal goals will influence the duration of the hypnotherapy sessions as well as the number of total sessions that you may need. Most people begin to see results in as few as two to four sessions.

DIY Hypnotherapy

If you are not comfortable working with a professional hypnotherapist or you can't afford the sessions, you can choose to perform self-hypnosis. While this is not as effective as the sessions under a professional, you can still try it and see if it can help you with your weight loss goals.

Here are the steps if you wish to practice self-hypnosis:

Believe in the power of hypnotism. Remember, this alternative treatment requires the person to be open and willing. It will not work for you if your mind is already set against it.

Find a comfortable and quiet room to practice hypnotherapy. Ideally, you should find a place that is free from noise and where no one can disturb you. Wear loose clothes and set relaxing music to help in setting up the mood.

Find a focal point. Choose an object in a room that you can focus on. Use your concentration on this object so you can start clearing your mind of all thoughts.

Breathe deeply. Start with five deep breaths, inhaling through your nose and exhaling through your mouth.

Close your eyes. Think about your eyelids becoming heavy and just let them close slowly.

Imagine that all stress and tension are coming out of your body. Let this feeling move down from your head, to your shoulders, to your chest, to your arms, to your stomach, to your legs, and finally to your feet.

Clear your mind. When you are relaxed, your account must be clear, and you can initiate the process of self-hypnotism.

Visualize a pendulum. In your mind, picture a moving swing. The movement of the pendulum is popular imagery used in hypnotism to encourage focus.

Start visualizing your ideal body image and size. This should help you instil in your subconscious the importance of healthy diet and exercise.

Suggest to yourself to avoid unhealthy food and start exercising regularly. You can use a particular mantra such as "I will exercise at least three times a week. Unhealthy food will make me sick."

Wake up. Once you have achieved what you want during hypnosis, you must wake yourself. Start by counting back from one to 10, and wake up when you reach 10.

Remember, a healthy diet doesn't mean that you have to reduce your food intake significantly. Just cut your consumption of food that is not healthy for you. Never hypnotize yourself out of eating. Only suggest to yourself to eat less of the food that you know is just making you fat.

Chapter 8
Hypnosis and Weight Loss

Hypnosis plays a vital role in medicinal solutions. In modern-day society, it is recommended for treating many different conditions, including obesity or weight loss in individuals who are overweight. It also serves patients who have undergone surgery exceptionally well, mainly if they are restricted from exercising after surgery. Given that it is the perfect option for losing weight, it is additionally helpful to anyone who is disabled or recovering from an injury.

Once you understand the practice and how it is conducted, you will find that everything makes sense. Hypnosis works for weight loss because of the relationship between our minds and bodies. Without proper communication being relayed from our minds to our bodies, we would not be able to function correctly. Since hypnosis allows the brain to adopt new ideas and habits, it can help push anyone in the right direction and could potentially improve our quality of living.

Adopting new habits can help eliminate fear, improve confidence, and inspire you to maintain persistence and a sense of motivation on your weight loss journey. Since two of the most significant issue's society faces today are media-based influences and a lack of motivation, you can quickly solve any problems related by merely correcting your mind.

Correcting your mind is an entirely different mission on its own, or without hypnosis, that is. It is a challenge that most will get frustrated. Nobody wants to deal with themselves. Although that may be true, perhaps one of the best lessons hypnosis teaches you is the significance of spending time focusing on your intentions. Daily practicing of hypnosis includes focusing on specific ideas. Once these ideas are normalized in your daily routine and life, you will find it easier to cope with struggles and ultimately break bad habits, which is the ultimate goal.

In reality, it takes 21 consecutive days to break a bad habit, but only if a person remains persistent, integrating both a conscious and consistent effort to quit or rectify a practice. It takes the same amount of time to adopt a new healthy habit. With hypnosis, it can take up to three months to either break a bad habit or form a new one. However, even though hypnosis takes longer, it tends to work far more effectively than just forcing yourself to do something you don't want to do.

Our brains are robust operating systems that can be fooled under the right circumstances. Hypnosis has been proven to be useful for breaking habits and adopting new ones due to its powerful effect on the mind. It can be measured in the same line of consistency and power as affirmations. Now, many would argue that hypnosis is unnecessary and that completing a 90-day practice of hypnotherapy to change habits for weight loss is a complete waste of time. However, when you think about someone who needs to lose weight but can't seem to do it, then you might start reconsidering it as a helpful solution to the problem. It's no secret that the human brain requires far more than a little push or single affirmation to thrive. Looking at motivational video clips and reading quotes every day is great but is it helping you to move further than from A to B?

It's true that today, we are faced with a sense of rushing through life. Asking an obese or unhealthy individual why they gained weight, there's a certainty that you'll receive similar answers.

Could it be that no one has time to, for instance, cook or prep healthy meals, visit the gym or move their bodies? Apart from making up excuses as to why you can't do something, there's actual evidence hidden in the reasons why we sell ourselves short and opt for the easy way out.

Could it be that the majority of individuals have just become lazy?

Regardless of your excuses, reasons or inabilities, hypnosis debunks the idea that you have to go all out to get healthier. Losing weight to improve your physical appearance has always been a challenge, and although there is no easy way out, daily persistence and 10 to 60 minutes a day of practice could help you to lose weight. Not just that, but it can also restructure your brain and help you to develop better habits, which will guide you in experiencing a much more positive and sustainable means of living.

Regardless of the practice or routine, you follow at the end of the day, the principle of losing weight always remains the same. You have to follow a balanced diet in proportion with a sustainable exercise routine.

By not doing so is where most people tend to go wrong with their weight loss journeys. It doesn't matter whether it's a diet supplement, weight loss tea, or even hypnosis. Your diet and exercise routine still play an increasingly important role in losing weight and will be the number one factor that will help you to obtain permanent results. There's a lot of truth in the advice given that there aren't any quick fixes to help you lose weight faster than what's recommended. Usually, anything that promotes standard weight loss, which is generally about two to five pounds a week, depending on your current Body Mass Index (BMI), works no matter what it is. The trick to losing weight doesn't necessarily lie in what you do, but instead in how you do it.

When people start with hypnosis, they may be very likely to quit after a few days or weeks, as it may not seem useful or it isn't leading to any noticeable results.

Nevertheless, if you remain consistent with it, eat a balanced diet instead of crash dieting, and follow a simple exercise routine, then you will find that it has a lot more to offer you than just weight loss. Even though weight loss is the goal of this book, it's essential to keep in mind that lasting results don't occur overnight. There are no quick fixes, especially with hypnosis.

Adopting the practice, you will discover many benefits, yet two of the most important ones are healing and learning how to activate the fat burning process inside of your body.

Hypnosis is not a diet, nor is it a fast-track method to get you where you want to go. Instead, it is a tool used to help individuals reach their goals by implementing proper habits. These habits can help you achieve results by focusing on appropriate diet and exercise. Since psychological issues influence most weight-related issues, hypnosis acts as the perfect tool, laying a foundation for a healthy mind.

Hypnosis is not a type of mind control, yet it is designed to alter your mind by shifting your feelings toward liking something that you might have hated before, such as exercise or eating a balanced diet. The same goes for quitting sugar or binge eating. Hypnosis identifies the root of the issues you may be dealing with and works by rectifying it accordingly. Given that it changes your thought pattern, you may also experience a much calmer and relaxed approach to everything you do.

Hypnosis works by maintaining changes made in mind because of neuroplasticity. Consistent hypnotherapy sessions create new patterns in the brain that result in the creation of new habits. Since consistency is the number one key to losing weight, it acts as a solution to overcome barriers in your mind, which is something the majority of individuals struggle. Hypnosis can also provide you with many techniques to meet different goals, such as gastric band hypnosis, which works by limiting eating habits, causing you to refrain from overeating.

Chapter 9
Find Your Motivation

One of the tools that are powerful in creating a significant change in life is Motivation. Your Motivation is based on what you believe. And as you are probably aware, belief is scarcely based on your concrete reality. In essence, you think things because of how you see them, feel them, hear them, smell them, and so forth. You can program your mind by taking feelings from one of your experiences and connecting those feelings to a different experience. Let us look at how you can remain motivated to lose weight:

Establish where you are now

It would be best if you took a full-length picture of yourself at present as a push mechanism from your current position, as well as for comparison later on. Two primary factors are relevant to health. One is whether you like the image you see in the mirror, and the second is how you feel. Do you have the energy to do what you wish, and are you feeling strong enough?

- Explore your reasons for wanting to lose weight. These are what will keep you going even when you don't feel like it.
- Assess your eating habits and establish your reasons for overeating or indulging in the wrong foods.

· It is assumed that you have the desire to get healthier and lose weight. Here, you state clearly and positively to yourself what you want, and then decide that you will accomplish it with persistence. Use the self-hypnosis routine explained above to drive this point into your subconscious mind.

· Determine your Motivation for the desired results, and how you will know when you've accomplished the goal. How will you feel, what you will see, and what are you likely to hear when you achieve your goal.

· Devote the first session of self-hypnosis to making the ultimate decision about your weight. Note that you must never have any doubt in your mind about your challenge to lose weight. Plan your meals every day. Weigh yourself frequently to monitor your progress as well. However, do not be paranoid about weighing yourself as this can negatively affect your development.

· Repeat to yourself every day that you are getting to your ideal weight, that you've developed new, sensible eating habits, and that you are no longer prone to temptation.

· Think positively and provide positive affirmations in your self-induced hypnotic state.

Tweak Your Lifestyle

Every little thing counts. This lesson is essential to know if you want to lose weight and slim down. Making a few changes in your regular daily activities can help you burn more calories.

Walk more

Use the stairs instead of the escalator or elevator if you're going up or down a floor or two.

Park the car you use far away from your destination and walk the rest of the way. You can also walk briskly to burn more calories.

During your rest day, make it more active by taking your dog for a long walk in the park.

If you need to travel a few blocks, save gas and avoid traffic by walking. For greater distances, dust off that old bike and pedal your way to your destination.

Watch how and what you eat.

A big breakfast kicks your body into hyper metabolism mode so you should not skip the first meal of the day.

Brushing after a meal signals your brain that you've finished eating, making you crave less until your next scheduled meal.

If you need to get food from a restaurant, make your order to-go so you won't get tempted by their other offerings.

Plan your meals for the week, so you can count how many calories you are consuming in a day.

Make quick, healthy meals, so you save time. There are thousands of recipes out there. Do some research.

Eat inside a place with a table, not in your car. Drive-thru food is almost always greasy and full of unhealthy carbohydrates.

Put more leaves, like arugula and alfalfa sprouts on your meals to give you more fiber and make you eat less.

Order the smallest meal size if you need to eat fast food.

Start your meal with a vegetable salad. Dip the mixture into the dressing instead of pouring it on.

For a midnight snack, munch on protein bars or drink a glass of skim milk.

Eat before you go to the grocery to keep yourself from being tempted by food items that you don't plan to buy.

Clean out your pantry by taking out food items that won't help you with your fitness goals.

The whole idea in the tweaks mentioned is that you should eat less and move more.

Chapter 10
Accept Current Reality

Life is not fair; neither is it unfair. It just is. We can accept life as it comes, or we can keep fighting people and circumstances, which will only result in frustration and discontentment. It is part of human nature to seek justice and fairness. When something unfair happens to us, the amygdala and the primitive part of our brain that results in a fight or flight response is triggered. It results in fear or anger, therefore explaining why we feel these emotions whenever we witness unfair occurrences. It triggers such strong physical and emotional reactions that if one is not conscious, it may lead to actions that you may regret later.

Humans have developed a cortex (the thinking brain) around the amygdala, which should assist in thinking through our reactions before we respond. Neurologically, the thinking brain kicks in a few seconds after the amygdala. Therefore, we should not be too fast to respond with the first emotions felt but should take time to think through the feelings and come up with a logical course of action.

Generally, people respond to unfairness in three significant ways, either they try to control everything, or they worry excessively about everything or they walk the middle path. Worrying is not bad. But excessive worry or rumination drains your energy typically, increases your anxiety, and makes you feel helpless because your focus is on the problem leading to inaction.

On the other hand, control freaks try to control every aspect of the situation, micromanaging everyone and everything. This is futile because you cannot control everything. The middle path is the best way whereby worry is your initial reaction, but you follow it up with brainstorming for a solution and then taking action in this direction.

Some Things Are out of Your Control

Much as we would like to believe that we are in control, there are very many things that are out of our control. Generally, the only things we have control over are our actions and our attitudes. Your attitude is a result of your perception. People do not like to feel helpless in situations, and this often results in coping mechanisms to manage the feeling of helplessness. Some of these coping mechanisms are:

· Complaining. This is a widespread coping mechanism and is typically used when the person who feels like they have been wronged can't think of a way of solving the problem; therefore, the person looks for reassurance and sometimes pity from others.

Binging. From over-eating to over-consumption of media (TV, Social media, and books), some people try to cope with stress through over-consumption rather than taking decisive action.

Blaming and projecting. This is whereby someone decides to give the responsibility of the stress to someone else and to judge them as the guilty party.

Using excuses. Some people always try to explain away their mistakes as a way of alleviating guilt or blame. It is a way of rationalizing your decisions after you have done them.

While these coping mechanisms may relieve the feeling for some time, they are useless when it comes to solving the problem. That is why some habits are repeated over and over again rather than looking for solutions that would solve the problem once and for all. How a person reacts to a problem may be indicative of where their locus of control lies. A person with an internal locus of control does not need the approval of others to feel good about themselves, and therefore they are more willing to accept that they are in the wrong and take action.

Why We Try to Control Factors and Place Blame

Projecting or numbing our emotions is often much more relaxed than self-searching, and finding blame in our actions. No one likes to be wrong. We avoid feeling the uncomfortable emotions that accompany being wrong by numbing rather than evaluating what we did and taking action to correct ourselves. Blaming and using excuses take the blame from us, thereby making us feel good about ourselves. A 50-50 approach can help by accepting that both parties could have a share of the responsibility, therefore, alleviating part of the guilt without excusing the need for action

We expect life to be fair, and when it isn't, we want to find who is guilty and make them pay for it. In a sense, placing blame is a way of punishing the wrong party for what they have done. This makes sense considering we often believe that actions have consequences, and we feel that by taking the blame, then we must suffer the consequences of the action. This is the rationalization that often leads to mob justice. When an injustice occurs, a group of people gets angry and decides to find the cause of their anger so that they can make them pay for their actions.

When you consider that placing blame does not correct the mistake made as we cannot go back in time, we find it is easier to look for a solution than to take the role of judge and jury. This does not mean that crime should go unpunished, but that the punishment should be left to the authorities, not just anyone who feels wronged.

When we try to take control and to place blame, we feel safe. When you know who has made a mistake and is to blame, we can distinguish who is 'evil' and who is 'good.' This distinction leads us to pick a side, mostly the side that is fair and true. In a way, this makes us feel that we are good people, and we are safe because the guilty side is made up of evil people. This distinction is, however, wrong because nobody is perfect, and making a mistake won't make you a wrong person any more than being on the right side will make you a saint. We should always be objective and not try to bring in our moral judgments when mistakes occur.

Blaming creates biases that affect perceptions. As human beings, we like attributing outcomes to people and things. For many people, they attribute positive results to themselves (internal attributions), and they attribute adverse outcomes to external factors (external attributions). For example, passing an exam is attributed to our efforts and failure assigned to an unfair teacher or a hard exam. Another attribution error is moral luck, whereby a person is only wrong if their wrong actions lead to adverse outcomes.

Therefore, a person who ignores a traffic signal is considered less wrong if they do not cause an accident compared to one who causes an accident. Regardless of fault, however, perception leads us to rigid thinking as you often find you do not want to listen to the other party. Biases create blindsides in our view and reactions and should be avoided at all costs.

Blaming comes from having a perfectionist mindset. This can be significantly attributed to social media as people ruthlessly edit how they appear, so they seem perfect but rarely want to show their struggles. When we blame, we do not want to look like we make mistakes in front of people because we assume that people will love us more if we are flawless. This is a fallacy because nobody is perfect and we all make mistakes. We will only experience real connections with other people when we are willing to be our authentic selves and show that we are fallible, and it is okay.

Blame excuses us from negative behavior and outcomes. If you fail a particular exam, the easy way out is to blame the teacher, the exam, or anything else but yourself. This is because the emotions that are associated with this failure, i.e., frustration and guilt, are not easy to bear. However, when you refuse to take responsibility, you also prevent yourself from learning the lesson, you were supposed to learn from the situation. After all, it is not failing. That is not the problem, but quitting is. Do not let your failures deter you from trying again. Be willing to learn the lesson failure is teaching you so that you do not fail in the same way again.

No matter how much we desire to control situations in our lives, we need to understand that there are some aspects of life that we will never be able to control. The following aspects can be considered:

· You cannot manage natural disasters and tragedies. It is futile to fight nature and life as you will always lose.

· You cannot control the actions that happened in the past. No amount of wishing, hoping, or praying will change past events.

· You cannot guarantee outcomes. You can do your best to try and get the best possible results, but beyond that, you have to let them be.

· You cannot change someone's decisions and behaviors. While you can advise them, it is always up to the person to change these things.

Blame vs. Responsibility

Placing blame is always the most natural way out of a situation. However, it doesn't solve the problem at hand. The best strategy is always to take responsibility, and this is always really hard to do. We may break down the word responsibility into two words, ability and response. Responsibility is, therefore, the ability to respond to a situation, so unlike blame, which is always looking to the past, responsibility is always looking to the future. It is always better to take responsibility because no amount of blame can correct a situation. So rather than ask 'who did this?' or 'why did you do this?' the wiser question is 'what can we do to make this better.' Remember that personal responsibility is a choice. You cannot force it on someone else.

There are many benefits to taking responsibility. They include:

· Taking responsibility always leads to a fast resolution of problems compared to having to sift through witness accounts to find who is responsible for what.

· Taking responsibility takes away the feeling of helplessness and instead offers us the opportunity to correct the situation.

· Taking responsibility allows us to practice empathy and compassion rather than taking a judgmental stance.

· Taking responsibility puts you firmly in the driver's seat of your life. Rather than letting your emotions and situations control your reactions, you choose to take control of your reactions.

· Taking responsibility allows us to assess ourselves and therefore leads us to learn from our mistakes.

How can you take responsibility?

· Determine the areas of your life that you can control and take action on these. Learn to accept the things that you cannot control.

· Remind yourself that outcomes are a result of the event and your response. Learn to recognize and differentiate responses that lead to positive outcomes and those that lead to adverse outcomes.

· Learn to differentiate between ruminating and problem-solving. Worry feeds itself, leading to more worry, but problem-solving leads you to solutions and is a more productive use of your time.

· Plan for stress management. Have strategies ready for when you feel stressed so that you know correctly what to do when you feel those uncomfortable emotions rising, for example, positive affirmations.

· Become more aware of your fears and emotions. Sometimes you realize that what you fear will happen when you take responsibility is not as bad as you think, and you can overcome it.

Concentrate on your circle of influence. Do not get caught up needlessly worrying about things that you know you cannot influence. An example of things you can't influence is natural disasters.

The life you want will come as a result of the choices you make. Don't allow life's circumstances to dictate and control your emotions. Don't give away your power by assigning blame in situations that you can easily take responsibility and resolve. The difference between victims and victors is in how they respond to the challenges they encounter.

Chapter 11
The Power of Guided Meditation

When you want to find ways to meditate calmly, you can try your hand at some other techniques that are designed to help you focus and settle your thoughts. One of the best methods to clear your head is to use your mantras or your affirmations in mantra meditation.

Find a comfortable place to sit, and rest yourself cross-legged with your hands on your knees. Try to keep your spine straight, as slumping is a posture of defeat, and you want to keep an aura of confidence. Choose a mantra to recite in your head, or try to recite your affirmation if it's not too long.

Close your eyes and try to imagine a candle burning. Focus on the flame as you slowly inhale and exhale. Essential yoga breathing works well for this meditation method. As you inhale, keep your mind's eye on the flame. As you exhale, think about your mantra, reciting it in your head or aloud. You can also use your goals or your milestones as your recitation. For example, if you are nearing a landmark in your weight loss plan, try using it during your meditation, like this:

Inhale, focused on the flame…

Exhale, say, "I'll hit my ten-pound mark this week."

Continue this exercise until you find your concentration flagging. You may need to start slow, working in five-minute increments, until you can meditate for a more extended, more effective period. Every little bit counts when it comes to mantra meditation.

Another active meditation for focus is a practice known as gazing. This technique is performed by choosing an object to study carefully and giving it your full attention until it's the only thing you are thinking about. Find your object and either hold it if it's small enough or sit near it if it's too large to hold. Trinkets like jewelry work for this meditation, as do simple pieces of artwork or an interesting article of clothing like a patterned scarf.

Sitting comfortably, use yoga breathing to calm yourself down, then begin to look at your object. You want to observe all its apparent qualities, beginning with things like colour and shape. Continue your observations, asking yourself, what does it feel like? Is it light or heavy? Take in all the physical properties of your chosen object. Think about the texture of the materials and the way the light reflects off of it. You want the only thing in the world to be the object in your gaze. Try not to look away; breaking your gaze will break the meditation. When you can no longer find anything new to observe about the object, close your eyes, and describe it to yourself. When you've finished, take a few deep breaths and open your eyes.

The idea behind gazing is to be able to concentrate all your energy on one goal- to keep your eyes on the prize literally. When you can use gazing as an active meditation, you will learn to build stamina and focus, which will help you further your weight loss goals, and in fact, any other goals you should choose to set for yourself.

Another great way to meditate quietly is to make a recording and play it back to yourself while you focus on your own words. Self-guided meditation is a beautiful way to lift yourself and remind yourself of your accomplishments thus far. You can use the voice recorder or video recorder application on your phone or a small digital recorder like a reporter might use for interviews. It takes little work, but write yourself a short script or some notes, and make a positive soundtrack for yourself.

You can record yourself talking over a backdrop of soothing music, with breaks in between so the tune can relax you as well. Aim for recording time of five to ten minutes, even if you only speak for a few minutes, and you edit a loop. Read your affirmation to yourself, calmly recite your mantras, or just give yourself a low-key pep talk. When it's time to meditate, find a comfy place to sit, take a few deep breaths, pop in your earphones, and press play. Focus on your own words lifting you to your next goal; it will do you a world of good as you move to your next milestone.

With all these meditation techniques to choose from, you may be thinking we're running out of methods to talk about, but we haven't even gotten to mindfulness yet! Meditation and mindfulness aren't the same, but they are allies to each other and you as you seek to lose weight and achieve a healthier lifestyle. Let's keep moving and see what mindfulness can do for you.

Chapter 12
The Power of Affirmations

Today is another day. Today is a day for you to start making a euphoric, satisfying life. Today is the day to begin to discharge every one of your impediments. Today is the day for you to get familiar with the privileged insights of life. You can transform yourself into improving things. You, as of now, include the devices inside you to do as such. These devices are your considerations and your convictions.

What Are Positive Affirmations?

For those of you who aren't acquainted with the advantages of positive affirmations, I'd prefer to clarify a little about them. A statement is genuinely anything you state or think. A great deal of what we typically report and believe is very harmful and doesn't make great encounters for us. We need to retrain our reasoning and to talk into positive examples if we need to change us completely.

An affirmation opens the entryway. It's a starting point on the way to change. When I talk about doing affirmations, I mean deliberately picking words that will either help take out something from your life or help make something new in your life.

Each idea you think and each word you express is an affirmation. The entirety of our self-talk, our interior exchange, is a flood of oaths. You're utilizing statements each second, whether you know it or not. You're insisting and making your background with each word and thought.

Your convictions are just routine reasoning examples that you learned as a youngster. The vast numbers of them work very well for you. Different beliefs might be restricting your capacity to make the very things you state you need. What you need and what you trust your merit might be unusual. You have to focus on your contemplations with the goal that you can start to dispose of the ones making encounters you don't need in your life.

It would help if you understood that each grievance is an affirmation of something you figure you don't need in your life. Each time you blow up, you're asserting that you need more annoyance in your life. Each time you feel like a casualty, you're confirming that you need to keep on feeling like a casualty. If you believe that you think that life isn't giving you what you need in your reality, at that point, it's sure that you will never have the treats that experience provides for others-that is, until you change how you think and talk.

You're not a terrible individual for intuition, how you do. You've quite recently never figured out how to think and talk. Individuals all through the world are quite recently starting to discover that our contemplations make our encounters. Your folks most likely didn't have the foggiest idea about this, so they couldn't in any way, shape, or form instruct it to you. They showed you what to look like at life in the manner that their folks told them. So no one isn't right. In any case, it's the ideal opportunity for us all to wake up and start to deliberately make our lives in a manner that satisfies and bolsters us. You can do it. I can do it. We, as a whole, can do it-we need to figure out how. So how about we get to it.

I'll talk about affirmations as a rule, and afterwards, I'll get too specific everyday issues and tell you the best way to roll out positive improvements in your wellbeing, your funds, your affection life, etc. Once you figure out how to utilize affirmations, at that point, you can apply the standards in all circumstances. A few people say that "affirmations don't work" (which is an affirmation in itself) when what they mean is that they don't have a clue how to utilize them accurately. Some of the time, individuals will say their affirmations once per day and gripe the remainder of the time. It will require some investment for affirmations to work if they're done that way. The grumbling affirmations will consistently win, because there is a higher amount of them, and they're generally said with extraordinary inclination.

In any case, saying affirmations is just a piece of the procedure. What you wrap up of the day and night is significantly progressively significant. The key to having your statements work rapidly and reliably is to set up air for them to develop in. Affirmations resemble seeds planted in soil: poor soil, poor development. Fertile soil, bottomless event. The more you decide to think contemplations that cause you to feel great, the faster the affirmations work.

So think upbeat musings, it's that straightforward. What's more, it is feasible. How you decide to believe, at present, is an only that-a decision. You may not understand it since you've thought along these lines for such a long time, yet it truly is a decision. Presently, today, this second, you can decide to change your reasoning. Your life won't pivot for the time being. Yet, in case you're reliable and settle on the decision regularly to think considerations that cause you to feel great, you'll unquestionably roll out positive improvements in each part of your life.

Positive Affirmations and How to Use Them

Positive affirmations are positive articulations that depict an ideal circumstance, propensity, or objective that you need to accomplish. Rehashing regularly these positive explanations, influences the psyche brain profoundly, and triggers it without hesitation, to bring what you are reworking into the real world.

The demonstration of rehashing the affirmations, intellectually or so anyone might hear, inspires the individual reworking them, builds the desire and inspiration, and pulls in open doors for development and achievement.

This demonstration likewise programs the psyche to act as per the rehashed words, setting off the inner mind-brain to take a shot at one's sake, to offer the positive expressions materialize.

Affirmations are extremely valuable for building new propensities, rolling out positive improvements throughout one's life, and for accomplishing objectives.

Affirmations help in weight misfortune, getting progressively engaged, concentrating better, changing propensities, and accomplishing dreams.

They can be helpful in sports, in business, improving one's wellbeing, weight training, and in numerous different zones.

These positive articulations influence in a proper manner, the body, the brain, and one's sentiments

Rehashing affirmations is very reasonable. Despite this, a lot of people do not know about this truth. Individuals, for the most part, restate negative statements, not positive ones. This is called negative self-talk.

On the off chance that you have been disclosing to yourself how miserable you can't contemplate, need more cash, or how troublesome life is, you have been rehashing negative affirmations.

Along these lines, you make more challenges and more issues, since you are concentrating on the problems, and in this way, expanding them, rather than concentrating on the arrangements.

A great many people rehash in their psyches pessimistic words and proclamations concerning the contrary circumstances and occasions in their lives, and therefore, make progressively bothersome circumstances.

Words work in two different ways, to assemble or obliterate. It is how we use them that decides if they will bring tremendous or destructive outcomes.

Affirmations in Modern Times

It is said that the French analyst and drug specialist Emile Coue is the individual who carried this subject to the open's consideration in the mid-twentieth century.

Emile Coue saw that when he told his patients how viable an elixir was, the outcomes were superior to if he didn't utter a word. He understood that musings that consume our psyches become a reality and that rehashing concepts and considerations is a sort of autosuggestion.

Emile Coue is associated with his acclaimed proclamation, "Consistently, all around, I am showing signs of improvement and better."

Later in the twentieth century, this was Louise Hay, who concentrated on this point and called autosuggestions – affirmations.

Chapter 13
How to Use Meditation and Affirmations to Lose Weight

No Nonsense Weight loss affirmations the loss of weight is a great goal, but it sure helps you to get where you want to go if you have affirmations of weight loss. So why do weight claims help you get where you want to go?

AFFIRMATION

Affirmations would help to wrap the mind around your goals and keep you focused as to where you want to be. So, when you're in its match, let's get those things moving.

Objective 1: Create the perfect healthy weight. The first bad part is to go there and achieve a certain ideal healthy weight. Don't talk about this. Even talk to your doctor about your ideal healthy level and do research. It is essential to raise an important subject at this stage. What is your ideal healthy weight, and assume you can't get there? It is safe to say that when it comes to appearance and obesity, society has set some rather strict standards.

When you see it, it is quite simple to define morbid obesity. This applies to a person who struggles with everyday life while carrying out basic tasks. But what happens to all of us if these tables that describe the criteria for the ideal height, weight, and body mass index of an individual cannot be matched? What are the rules if you are too thin?

Especially if you're not fit, there is a risk of being too thin. It would be far safer to be slightly overweight, but fit and healthy according to the scale. So, use common sense and never set your ideal weight by guess or because you think that this is the only weight you can take pleasure in. Focus your ideal weight on being healthy, but above all, a weight to keep you active and fit.

Objective 2: How I Am Going to Finish Objective 1.

You have your ideal healthy weight established, and you need to get there now. It's just another wasted opportunity if you don't. Next, ignore the lazy diet pills and crash diets that will take you back to where you started or worse. How is this a positive statement? See a fat farmer ever? I say one who works the farm every day. What makes the difference? The right to eat and physical activity. The body is designed for frequent and varied exercises. The main components of Objective 2 must be both aerobic and motivational tasks. For food, a balanced diet should be consumed, which takes approximately 1800-2800 calories a day for one person and less for a woman. Include as much organic food as possible to avoid fast food and processed food. Eat vegetables and fruits.

Objective #3-Believe it!

All right, we have Target 1 and Target 2 planned, now how can we convince ourselves that we're going to achieve these without falling off the car? You've been happy to ask about this. First, why do I have to believe it? Can I not just go?

Ever hear the phrase "been there"? That could only be the case, and how did it work? Not too good, perhaps, or you wouldn't be here now.

Meet your new best friend to help you with the third objective. The meaning of these words your head doesn't know: I can't, I won't give up, forget about it, or, "Let's go to the Dairy Queen," most statements are more likely to finish when they're written. Detail how your life has changed by eating better, looking better, and feeling better. Talk about where you began and how you took a step closer to achieving goal #1 each day. Talk about how you might be tempted to give up, but here you remembered, saying NOT TODAY OR EVER!! And finally, when you reach your goal, how proud you are and how you don't go the old way or weight.

Objective 4-Remember that you have your head into the game every day for goal #3. Okay, you've got to keep it in the game. How? By confirming your stated Objectives #1 to #3. You likely have to hear them out once a day so that you don't forget them. Once you free your mind, there's a saying that your rear end will lead. Hold with your head your body parts in the game.

Here are your claims of weight loss: plan it wisely, change the lifestyle, enter the game, and bring your body with you. Continue to talk to yourself because you are your best friend. This must not be torture. Take joy in the fact that the reward you want and deserve is your path.

MEDITATION

Meditation has long been recognized as the tested path to self-improvement, the ratings of which are very high because it involves only sitting there and holding your inner self and being at peace with yourself. It's an excellent way to change your life.

Self-esteem is one field that benefits significantly from the practice of the art of meditation. It refers to the way people view themselves, which also describes how self-confidence is nurtured.

It is believed that a daily dose of meditation will help to remove the illusion that you may have about yourself because what you are is only about how you project your image. Meditation is going to help you realize who you are.

If you have a complex of inferiority or don't think about yourself very much, it means you need to improve your image. That's where easy meditation will help you make things better; it's necessary to do your morning and evening routine. It's going to make you think better and calmer.

It is the pillar of self-esteem because it will help you have peace within yourself and increase your faith in life.

You will start interacting with people in a better way with your renewed confidence and face things with greater confidence without relying on any other support to make you feel secure.

No more pretense or attempt to pass as a character you're not going to be. This means you're going to be more comfortable and not concerned about life anymore. You're just going to relax and let life stuff take its course.

What you're going to do is take a little time every morning and night, spend no less than 30 minutes of meditation a day. You will see things start to change within two weeks or a month if you continue to do this.

Chapter 14
Guided Meditation for Weight Loss

Before you can begin using meditations to do things such as help you burn fat, you need to make sure that you set yourself up correctly for your meditation sessions. Each meditation is going to consist of you entering a deep state of relaxation, following guided hypnosis, and then awakening yourself out of this state of relaxation. If done correctly, you will find yourself experiencing the stages of changed mindset and changed behavior that follows the session.

To properly set yourself up for a meditation experience, you need to make sure that you have a quiet space where you can engage in your meditation. You want to be as uninterrupted as possible so that you do not stir awake from your meditation session. Aside from having a quiet space, you should also make sure that you are comfortable in the area that you will be in. For some of the meditations, I will share, you can be lying down or doing this meditation before bed so that the information sinks in as you sleep. For others, you are going to want to be sitting upright, ideally with your legs crossed on the floor, or with your feet planted on the floor as you sit in a chair. Staying in a sitting position, especially during morning meditations, will help you stay awake and increase your motivation. Laying down during these meditations earlier in the day may result in you draining your energy and feeling completely exhausted, rather than motivated. As a result, you may work against what you are trying to achieve.

Each of these meditations is going to involve a visualization practice; however, if you find that visualization is generally difficult for you, you can listen. The key here is to make sure that you keep as open of a mind as possible so that you can stay receptive to the information coming through these guided meditations.

Aside from all of the above, listening to low music, using a pillow or a small blanket, and dressing in comfortable loose clothing will all help you have better meditations. You want to make sure that you make these experiences the best possible so that you look forward to them and regularly engage in them. As well, the more relaxed and comfortable you are, the more receptive you will be to the information being provided to you within each meditation.

A Simple Daily Weight Loss Meditation

This meditation is an excellent simple meditation for you to use daily. It is a short meditation that will not take more than about 15 minutes to complete, and it will provide you with excellent motivation to stick to your weight loss regimen every single day. You should schedule time in your morning routine to engage in this simple daily weight loss meditation every single day. You can also complete it periodically throughout the day if you find your motivation dwindling or your mindset regressing. Over time, you should find that using it just once per day is plenty.

Because you are using this medication in the morning, make sure that you are sitting upright with a straight spine so that you can stay engaged and awake throughout the entire meditation. Laying down or getting too comfortable may result in you feeling more tired, rather than more awake, from your meditation. Ideally, this meditation should lead to boosted energy as well as improved fat burning abilities within your body.

The Meditation

Start by gently closing your eyes and drawing your attention to your breath. As you do, I want you to track the next five breaths, gently and intentionally lengthening them to help you relax as deeply as you can. With each breath, breathe into the count of five and out to the count of seven. Starting with your next breath in, 1, 2, 3, 4, 5, and out, 1, 2, 3, 4, 5, 6, and 7. Again, 1, 2, 3, 4, 5, and out, 1, 2, 3, 4, 5, 6, 7. Breathe in, 1, 2, 3, 4, 5, and breathe out, 1, 2, 3, 4, 5, 6, and 7. Again, breathe in, 1, 2, 3, 4, 5, and breathe out, 1, 2, 3, 4, 5, 6, and 7. One more time, breathe in, 1, 2, 3, 4, 5, and breathe out, 1, 2, 3, 4, 5, 6, and 7.

Now that you are starting to feel more relaxed, I want you to draw your awareness into your body. First, become aware of your feet. Feel your feet relaxing deeply, as you visualize any stress or worry melting away from your feet. Now, become aware of your legs. Feel any stress or worry melting away from your legs as they begin to relax completely. Next, become aware of your glutes and pelvis, allowing any stress or worry to fade away as they completely relax. Now, relax your entire torso, allowing any stress or anxiety to melt away from your body as it relaxes completely. Next, become aware of your shoulders, arms, hands, and fingers. Allow the stress and worry to melt away from your shoulders, arms, hands, and fingers as they relax entirely. Now, let the stress and fear melt away from your neck, head, and face. Feel your neck, head, and face relaxing as any stress or anxiety melts away completely.

As you deepen into this state of relaxation, I want you to take a moment to visualize the space in front of you. Imagine that in front of you, you are standing there looking back at yourself. See every inch of your body as it is right now standing before you, casually, as you observe yourself. While you do, see what parts of your body you want to reduce fat in so that you can create a healthier, more muscular body for yourself. Visualize the fat in these areas of your body, slowly fading away as you begin to carve out a more robust, leaner, and more muscular body underneath. Notice how effortlessly this extra fat melts away as you continue to visualize yourself becoming a healthier and more animated version of yourself.

Now, I want you to visualize what this healthier, leaner version of yourself would be doing. Visualize yourself going through your typical daily routine, except the perspective of your healthier self. What would you be eating? When and how would you be exercising? What would you spend your time doing? How do you feel about yourself? How different do you feel when you interact with the people around you, such as your family and your co-workers? What does life feel like when you are a healthier, leaner version of you?

Spend several minutes visualizing how different your life is now that your fat has melted away. Feel how natural it is for you to enjoy these healthier foods, and how easy it is for you to moderate your cravings and indulgences when you choose to treat yourself. Notice how easy it is for you to engage in exercise and how exercise feels enjoyable and like a beautiful hobby, rather than a chore that you have to force yourself to commit to every single day. Feel yourself genuinely enjoying life far more, all because the unhealthy fats that were weighing you down and disrupting your health have faded away. Notice how easy it was for you to get here, and how easy it is for you to continue to maintain your health and wellness as you continue to choose better and better choices for you and your body.

Feel how much you respect your body when you make these healthier choices, and how much you genuinely care about yourself. Notice how each meal and each exercise feels like an act of self-care, rather than a chore you are forcing yourself to engage in. Feel how good it feels to do something for you and your wellbeing.

When you are ready, take that visualization of yourself and send the image out far, watching it become nothing more than a spec in your field of awareness. Then, send it out into the ether, trusting that your subconscious mind will hold onto this vision of yourself and work daily on bringing this version of you into your current reality.

Now, awaken back into your body where you sit right now. Feel yourself feeling more motivated, more energized, and more excited about engaging in the activities that are going to improve your health and help you burn your fat. As you prepare to go about your day, hold onto that visualization and those feelings that you had of yourself, and trust that you can have this enjoyable experience in your life. You can do it!

Chapter 15

100 Positive Affirmations for Weight Loss

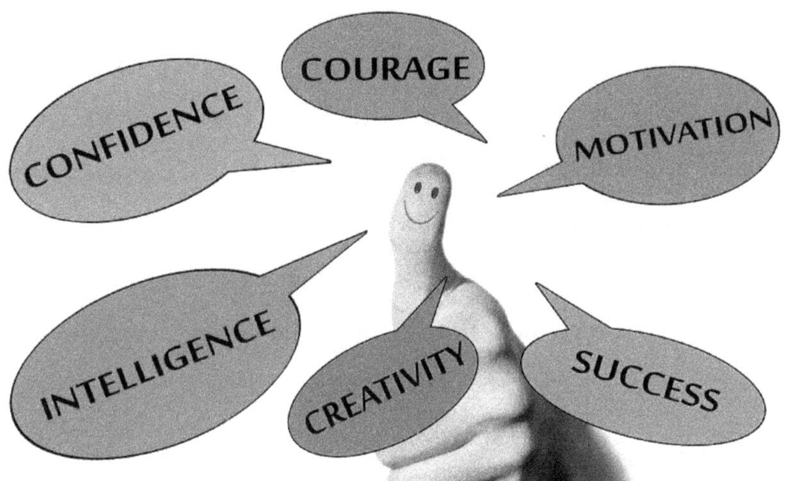

George taught Bonnie a hundred useful positive affirmations for weight loss and to keep her motivated. She chose the ones that she wanted to build in her program and used them every day. Bonnie was losing weight very slowly, which bothered her very much. She thought she was going in the wrong direction and was about to give up, but George told her not to worry because it was a completely natural speed. It takes time for the subconscious to collate all the information and start working according to her conscious will. Besides, her body remembered the fast weight loss, but her subconscious remembered her emotional damage, and now it is trying to prevent it. In reality, after some months of hard work, she started to see the desired results. She weighed 74 kilos (163 lbs.).

***

According to dietitians, the success of dieting is greatly influenced by how people talk about lifestyle changes for others and themselves.

The use of "I should" or "I must" is to avoid whenever possible. Anyone who says, "I shouldn't eat French fries" or "I have to get a bite of chocolate" will feel that they have no control over the events. Instead, if you say "I prefer" to leave the food, you will feel more power and less guilt. The term "dieting" should be avoided. Proper nutrition is s as a permanent lifestyle change. For example, the correct wording is, "I've changed my eating habits" or "I'm eating healthier".

Diets are fattening. Why?

The body needs fat. Our body wants to live, so it stores fat. Removing this amount of fat from the body is not an easy task as the body protects against weight loss. During starvation, our bodies switch to a 'saving flame', burning fewer calories to avoid starving. Those who are starting to lose weight are usually optimistic, as, during the first week, they may experience 1-3 kg (2-7 lbs.) of weight loss, which validates their efforts and suffering. Their body, however, has deceived them very well because it actually does not want to break down fat. Instead, it begins to break down muscle tissue. At the beginning of dieting, our bodies burn sugar and protein, not fat. Burned sugar removes a lot of water out of the body; that's why we experience amazing results on the scale. It should take about seven days for our body to switch to fat burning. Then our body's alarm bell rings. Most diets have a sad end: reducing your metabolic rate to a lower level-- Meaning, that if you only eat a little more afterwards, you regain all the weight you have lost previously. After dieting, the body will make special efforts to store fat for the next impending famine. What to do to prevent such a situation?

We must understand what our soul needs. Those who really desire to have success must first and foremost change their spiritual foundation. It is important to pamper our souls during a period of weight loss. All overweight people tend to rag on themselves for eating forbidden food, "I overate again. My willpower is so weak!" If you have ever tried to lose weight, you know these thoughts very well.

Imagine a person very close to you who has gone through a difficult time while making mistakes from time to time. Are we going to scold or try to help and motivate them? If we really love them, we would instead comfort them and try to convince them to continue. No one tells their best friend that they are weak, ugly, or bad, just because they are struggling with their weight. If you wouldn't say it to your friend, don't do so to yourself either! Let us be aware of this: during weight loss, our soul needs peace and support. Realistic thinking is more useful than disaster theory. If you are generally a healthy consumer, eat some goodies sometimes because of its delicious taste and to pamper your soul.

I'll give you a list of a hundred positive affirmations you can use to reinforce your weight loss. I'll divide them into main categories based on the most typical situations for which you would need confirmation. You can repeat all of them whenever you need to, but you can also choose the ones that are more suitable for your circumstances. If you prefer to listen to them during meditation, you can record them with a piece of sweet relaxing music in the background.

General affirmations to reinforce your wellbeing:

1. I'm grateful that I woke up today. Thank you for making me happy today.

2. Today is a perfect day. I meet friendly and helpful people, whom I treat kindly.

3. Every new day is for me. I live to make myself feel good. Today I just pick good thoughts for myself.

4. Something wonderful is happening to me today.

5. I feel good.

6. I am calm, energetic and cheerful.

7. My organs are healthy.

8. I am satisfied and balanced.

9. I live in peace and understanding with everyone.

10. I listen to others with patience.

11. In every situation, I find the good.

12. I accept and respect myself and my fellow human beings.

13. I trust myself; I trust my inner wisdom.

Do you often scold yourself? Then repeat the following affirmations frequently:

14. I forgive myself.

15. I'm good to myself.

16. I motivate myself over and over again.

17. I'm doing my job well.

18. I care about myself.

19. I am doing my best.

20. I am proud of myself for my achievements.

21. I am aware that sometimes I have to pamper my soul.

22. I remember that I did a great job this week.

23. I deserved this small piece of candy.

24. I let go of the feeling of guilt.

25. I release the blame.

26. Everyone is imperfect. I accept that I am too.

If you feel pain when you choose to avoid delicious food, then you need to motivate yourself with affirmations such as:

27. I am motivated and persistent.

28. I control my life and my weight.

29. I'm ready to change my life.

30. Changes make me feel better.

31. I follow my diet with joy and cheerfulness.

32. I am aware of my amazing capacities.

33. I am grateful for my opportunities.

34. Today I'm excited to start a new diet.

35. I always keep in mind my goals.

36. I imagine myself slim and beautiful.

37. Today I am happy to have the opportunity to do what I have long been postponing.

38. I possess the energy and will to go through my diet.

39. I prefer to lose weight instead of wasting time on momentary pleasures.

Here you can find affirmations that help you to change harmful convictions and blockages:

40. I see my progress every day.

41. I listen to my body's messages.

42. I'm taking care of my health.

43. I eat healthy food.

44. I love who I am.

45. I love how life supports me.

46. A good parking space, coffee, conversation. It's all for me today.

47. It feels good to be awake because I can live in peace, health, love.

48. I'm grateful that I woke up. I take a deep breath of peace and tranquility.

49. I love my body. I love being served by me.

50. I eat by tasting every flavor of the food.

51. I am aware of the benefits of healthy food.

52. I enjoy eating healthy food and being fitter every day.

53. I feel energetic because I eat well.

Many people are struggling with being overweight because they don't move enough. The very root of this issue can be a refusal to do exercises due to negative biases in our minds.

We can overcome these beliefs by repeating the following affirmations:

54. I like moving because it helps my body burn fat.

55. Each time I exercise, I am getting closer to having a beautiful, tight shapely body.

56. It's a very uplifting feeling of being able to climb up to 100 steps without stopping.

57. It's easier to have an excellent quality of life if I move.

58. I like the feeling of returning to my home tired but happy after a long winter walk.

59. Physical exercises help me have a longer life.

60. I am proud to have better fitness and agility.

61. I feel happier thanks to the happiness hormone produced by exercise.

62. I feel full thanks to the enzymes that produce a sense of fullness during physical exercises.

63. I am aware even after exercise, my muscles continue to burn fat, and so I lose weight while resting.

64. I feel more energetic after exercises.

65. My goal is to lose weight; therefore, I exercise.

66. I am motivated to exercise every day.

67. I lose weight while I exercise.

Now, I am going to give you a list of generic affirmations that you can build in your program:

68. I'm glad I'm who I am.

69. Today, I read articles and watch movies that make me feel positive about my diet progress.

70. I love it when I'm happy.

71. I take a deep breath and exhale my fears.

72. Today I do not want to prove my truth, but I want to be happy.

73. I am strong and healthy. I'm fine, and I'm getting better.

74. I am happy today because whatever I do, I find joy in it.

75. I pay attention to what I can become.

76. I love myself and am helpful to others.

77. I accept what I cannot change.

78. I am happy that I can eat healthy food.

79. I am happy that I have been changing my life with my new healthy lifestyle.

80. Today I do not compare myself to others.

81. I accept and support who I am and turn to myself with love.

82. Today I can do anything for my improvement.

83. I'm fine. I'm happy for life. I love who I am. I'm strong and confident.

84. I am calm and satisfied.

85. Today is perfect for me to exercise and to be healthy.

86. I have decided to lose weight, and I am strong enough to follow my will.

87. I love myself, so I want to lose weight.

88. I am proud of myself because I follow my diet program.

89. I see how much stronger I am.

90. I know that I can do it.

91. It is not my past, but my present that defines me.

92. I am grateful for my life.

93. I am grateful for my body because it collaborates well with me.

94. Eating healthy foods supports me to get the best nutrients I need to be in the best shape.

95. I eat only healthy foods, and I avoid processed foods.

96. I can achieve my weight loss goals.

97. All cells in my body are fit and healthy, and so am I.

98. I enjoy staying healthy and sustaining my ideal weight.

99. I feel that my body is losing weight right now.

100. I care about my body by exercising every day.

Chapter 16
Heal your Relation with Food

A straightforward method to perform this is to keep a food journal and a mood journal. Write down each time you know you've consumed unhealthy foods. Look back later on what feelings make you eat. You'll be able to recognize patterns or beliefs that make you overeat as time goes by. When you know what is causing your emotional eating, you will start working on how to avoid it and find ways to eat healthier.

1. Find other ways to fuel your emotions.

When you can't find another way to deal with your feelings without requiring food, so breaking this practice would be almost impossible. One of the reasons diets fail is that they give rational nutrition recommendations under the premise that lack of awareness is the only thing that stops you from eating properly. That form of suggestion only works if you can control eating habits. It's not enough to recognize your causes and grasp your process to stop emotional eating — you need to find new ways to cope with your emotions. You can call or have a hangout with a friend who makes you feel better when you're depressed or lonely, visit places you like, read an interesting book, watch a comedy show or play with the cat.

2. When cravings arrive, pause.

This might not be as simple as it sounds, because it is all you might think about when the desire for the food hits. You feel right there, and then, the need to feed. Taking at least five minutes before you give up on the craving, this gives you time to think about the wrong decision you're about to make. You can change your mind within that time, and make a better choice. Start with 2 minutes if 5 minutes is a lot for you and increasing the time as you get better with it.

3. Learn to embrace good feelings and negative ones.

Emotional eating comes from being unable to cope with the feelings on the brain. Find a friend or therapist who will speak to you about the problems and concerns you have. Being willing to accept negative and good emotions without having to include food would improve change.

4. Commit to healthy lifestyle habits.

Exercise, rest and adequate sleep will make it easier for you to deal with any emotional or physical problem you may experience. Create time for at least five days a week for a 30-minute workout, relax, and sleep 7 to 8 hours a day. It's also essential to surround yourself with caring people who will empower you and help you cope with your issues.

The first thing to keep emotional eating in mind is the addictive effect food has on you. You may encounter cravings that often feel uncontrollable, and you may feel as though you are addicted to food much as a smoker is addicted to smoking. The trick is to properly control your emotions and feelings and train your brain not to respond to stressful or unpleasant feelings by merely having to eat food (your preference brain drug) to calm down.

There are a few other useful methods and approaches that you can use to avoid emotional eating and lose weight, including: abandon the Diet!

Dieting ruins your metabolism, and you can eventually find yourself taking on weight. In reality, dieting will only work in the short run and will lower your fragile self-esteem.

Adjust your way of thinking.

Don't equate to anyone.

When you lose weight, it is crucial not to equate your weight with the importance of those around you. If you're unhappy with your weight, comparing yourself to the skinny girls you see in magazines or on television could prolong your recovery process by adjusting your lifestyle habits with eating, exercise, and mind control; you'll find it much easier to stop emotional eating and lose the weight you want much faster and longer-term.

When you've mastered techniques for managing your eating causes, your emotional food cravings should cease.

In a person who is in control of their emotions and has more constructive ways of coping with negative feelings, emotional eating cannot thrive – it is unlikely. You can eat intuitively before you know it, and be free from raw food and excess body fat for good.

Over-food is still not given the due treatment it deserves. It is always seen as not a real issue and to be laughing at something. That view is entirely false because it is a horrific illness that needs urgent care. The positive news is that taking action to help yourself avoid emotional eating forever is easy to do. I say that because I did it myself.

Stage # 1-Identifying the causes.

For each person, emotional eating is caused differently. Some people get the cravings when stressed out, and some when depressed or bored. You have to think a bit to figure out what your emotional causes are. When you know what they are, you will be given early notice when the desire to eat comes upon you.

Step # 2-Eliminating Temptation.

The one thing many people don't know about emotional eating is that often the craving is for one particular food. It is mostly ice-cream or candy for kids. Usually, for people, it's pizza. If you couldn't satisfy this temptation, that's not going to bother you as much. Clear out any of these temptations from your house. Throw out any nearby pizza delivery places. Once you know your tempters, get rid of them and make overeating hard for you.

Step # 3-The link breaks.

When the impulse hits, it's intense and instant. You are now feeling like eating. Good! You need to break this immediate bond by giving yourself sometime between the desire and the eating to avoid this.

- Call a friend
- Count to 60
- Write down what you feel
- Do some exercises
- Go outside for a walk
- Take a shower.

Whatever you can do to let the urge subside do wonder. Take these three steps, and you'll be doing them easier early and conquer emotional eating for good.

Would you like to learn the best ideas on how emotional eating stops working? It's emotional eating that satisfies your sensitive appetite. It has nothing to do with your kitchen, but in your mind lies the issue. What are the most potent methods to overcome the emotional eating temptation? Make a list to relieve your cravings for food.

Prepare for future emotional eating issues. Draw a piece of paper and a pencil over the weekend and take a route about your activities in the days ahead. Your map will show the stops you intend to make and potential detours. Choose an icon that reflects emotional eating. Place the image over an occurrence or activity that could cause your cravings for food, like an early lunch with your in-laws. Prepare ahead for that case. Look for the restaurant menu online so you can order something delicious but still good.

Clear the fears inside out. It helps if you take a deep breath, anytime you are nervous. Another thing you should do is to do a visual trick to detoxify yourself from the stress. Breathe in deeply and imagine a squeegee put near your head (that piece of cloth you use to clean your window or windshield). Breathe out slowly, and believe the squeegee is wiping clean your heart. With it taking away all the worries. Do this quad.

Self-talk as if you're royalty. Usually, self-criticism goes to emotional eating. Toxic words you say to yourself, such as "I'm such a loser" or "I can't seem to be doing anything right", force you to drive to the closest. Don't be misled even though these claims are brief. Such feelings are like acid rain, which is slowly eroding your wellbeing. The next time you're caught telling yourself these negative words, counteracting by moving to a third-person perspective. In moments when you think "I'm such a mess", then remind yourself that "Janice is such a mess, but Janice will do what it takes to make it work out and make herself happy". This approach will help you out of the negative self-talk loop and give you some perspective. Pull up and be positive, and you'll have the strength to avoid emotional eating.

How can hypnosis aid with weight loss keep you stuck in a vicious cycle?

Hypnotherapy is aimed at improving your eating habits and increased levels of trust and encouragement to help you achieve success. There are six steps to the Goldcrest Hypnotherapy Weight Loss plan to be effective in losing weight for good:

1. Establish ATTITUDE ON RIGHT.

To lose weight, you must be inspired, determined and focused. Hypnotherapy can help you to be optimistic and to trust that you will lose weight and lead a healthier life. It should reframe your thoughts and empower you to take full responsibility for handling your pressure. Part of the hypnotherapy is to concentrate on the habits of self-defeating thinking that might have caused you to give up in the past.

2. No. Establish Habits, HEALTHY EATING.

If your mentality is right and fired up, I'll help you let go of the unhealthy eating habits and motivate you to lose weight by adopting healthy eating habits. The purpose is to help you regain control over food and increase your desire to lead a healthy life, including increased exercise wherever possible. The counselling should involve recognizing patterns of eating and seeking ways to improve eating habits. I'm going to help you build an eating plan that follows 80-20 law. You'll eat 80% of the time comfortably and have a bit of what you'd like for the remaining 20%.

3. Think about it. SET GOALS Low.

You may want to be the same size that you were when you were at college. But that could mean a five stone loss. Don't set such a big target for yourself. Divide the broad goal into smaller objectives. Set yourself 5 per cent or 10 per cent lower, more achievable targets and allow yourself a much longer timeline to accomplish it.

Giving yourself a bit of flexibility is also necessary. Your weight-loss journey will have ups and downs. It's essential your weight loss program is not static but flexible; otherwise, it won't feel like it suits into your life.

4. No. SET Target SPECIFIC.

Should not set common targets such as: "I have to consume less food" or "I have to do more".

Instead, set specific short-term goals such as: "I'm going to take a healthy lunch to work every day instead of going to a fast-food restaurant" or "I'm going to go on a Monday and Wednesday night after work every week for a 30-minute walk with my friend".

5. EAT BREAKFAST ALL TODAY.

Most people miss breakfast for being too busy or not hungry. Eat slow foods which release energy, such as oats, that will keep you going until lunch.

Set your alarm ahead of time. Make sure you go to bed 15 minutes sooner, so you don't cut down on your overall sleep.

6. As MINDFULLY EAT FOOD.

Learn to take your food in small bites. Slowly chew each mouthful, concentrating your attention on the food's texture, sounds and flavors.

To help you eat more slowly, place your cutlery between each mouthful. You should spend about 20 minutes eating every meal in a perfect world. Set a timer to help you adjust the time you're eating, so you know how long you've spent eating.

Chapter 17
How to Practice Every Day

Exercise Regularly

Exercise is good for human health in many ways, regardless of what you choose to do.

Although the DASH diet focuses on food choices, there is no denying that regular and varied exercise represents an essential component of a healthy lifestyle and one that can confer additional benefits.

With that said, the CDC identifies moderate-intensity aerobic activity that totals 120 to 150 minutes weekly, in combination with two additional weekly days of muscular resistance training, as an ideal combination to confer numerous health benefits to adults. Per the CDC, these benefits include the following:

Better weight management: When combined with dietary modification, regular physical activity plays a role in supporting or enhancing weight-management efforts. Regular exercise is a great way to expend calories on top of any dietary changes you will be making on this program.

Reduced risk for cardiovascular disease: A reduction in blood pressure is a well-recognized benefit of regular physical activity, which ultimately contributes to a reduced risk of cardiovascular disease.

Reduced risk of type 2 diabetes: Regular physical activity is known to improve blood glucose control and insulin sensitivity.

Improved mood: Regular physical activity is associated with improvements in mood and reductions in anxiety owing to how exercise positively influences the biochemistry of the human brain by releasing hormones and affecting neurotransmitters.

Better sleep: Those who exercise more regularly tend to sleep better than those who don't, which may be partly owing to the reductions in stress and anxiety that often occur in those who exercise regularly.

Stronger bones and muscles: Combining cardiovascular and resistance training confers severe benefits to both your bones and your muscles, which keep your body functioning at a high level as you age.

A longer life span: Those who exercise regularly tend to enjoy a lower risk of chronic disease and a longer life span.

As you will see in the 28-day plan, your recommended exercise totals will meet by exercising four out of the seven days a week. The exercise days will break up as follows: All four of the active days will include aerobic exercise for 30 minutes. As a beginner, I encourage you to start slowly and build up to four days. Two of the four active days will also include strength training. The bottom line is that you don't have to exercise for hours each day to enjoy the health benefits of physical activity. Our goal with this plan is to make the health benefits of exercise as accessible and attainable as possible for those who are ready and willing to give it a try.

Getting the Most Out of Your Workouts

Just as with healthy eating strategies, there are certain essential things to keep in mind about physical activity that will help support your long-term success. Let's take a look at a few crucial considerations that will help you get the most out of your workouts:

Rest days: Even though we haven't even started, I'm going to preach the importance of proper rest. Don't forget that you are taking part in this journey to improve your health for the long term, not to burn yourself out in 28 days. Although some of you with more experience with exercise may feel confident going above and beyond, my best advice for the majority of those reading is to listen to your body and take days off to minimize the risk of injury and burnout.

Stretching life: Stretching is a great way to prevent injury and keep you pain-free both during workouts and daily. Whether it's a planned activity after an exercise or through additional means such as yoga, stretching is beneficial in many ways.

Enjoyment: There is no right or wrong style of exercise. You are being provided with a different plan that emphasizes a variety of different cardiovascular and resistance training exercises. If there are certain activities within these groups that you don't enjoy, it's okay not to do them. Your ability to stick with regular physical activity in the long term will depend on finding a style of exercise that you enjoy.

Your limits: Physical activity is right for you, and it should be fun, too. It's up to you to keep it that way. While it is essential to challenge yourself, don't risk injury by taking things too far too fast.

Your progress: Although this is not an absolute requirement, some of you reading may find joy and fulfilment through tracking your exercise progress and striving toward a longer duration, more repetitions, and so on. If you are the type who enjoys a competitive edge, it may be fun to find a buddy to exercise and progress with.

Warm-ups: Last but certainly not least, your exercise routine will benefit significantly from a proper warm-up routine, which includes starting slowly or doing exercises similar to the ones included in your workout, but at a lower intensity.

Set a Routine

The exercise part of the DASH plan was developed with CDC exercise recommendations in mind to support your best health. For some, the 28-day policy may seem like a lot; for others, it may not seem like that much. If we look at any exercise routine from a very general perspective, there are at least three broad categories to be aware of.

Strength training: This involves utilizing your muscles against some form of counterweight, which may be your own body or dumbbells. These types of activities alter your resting metabolic rate by supporting the development of muscle while also strengthening your bones.

Aerobic exercise: Also known as a cardiovascular activity, these are the quintessential exercises such as jogging or running that involve getting your body moving and getting your heart rate up.

Mobility, flexibility, and balance: Stretching after workouts or even devoting your exercise time on one day a week to stretching or yoga is a great way to maintain mobility and prevent injury in the long term.

This routine recommends involving a combination of both cardiovascular and resistance training.

You will be provided with a wide array of options to choose from to accommodate a diverse exercise routine.

My best recommendation is to settle on the types of exercises that offer a balance between enjoyment and challenge. Remember that the benefits of physical activity are to be enjoyed well beyond just your 28-day plan, and the best way to ensure that is the case is selecting movements you genuinely enjoy.

Cardio and Body Weight Exercises

Cardio

Brisk walking: This is mainly walking at a pace beyond your standard walking rate for a purpose beyond just getting from point A to point B.

Jogging: This is the intermediary stage between brisk walking and running and can be used as an accompaniment to either exercise, depending on your fitness level.

Running: The quintessential and perhaps most well-recognized cardiovascular exercise.

Jumping jacks: Although 30 minutes straight of jumping jacks may be impractical, they are an excellent complement to the other activities on this list.

Dancing: Those who have a background in dancing may enjoy using it to their advantage, but anyone can put on their favorite songs and dance like nobody is watching.

Jump rope: Own a jump rope? Why not use it as part of your cardiovascular workout? It is a fun way to get your cardio in.

Other options (equipment permitting): Activities like rowing, swimming and water aerobics, biking, and using elliptical and stair climbing machines can be great ways to exercise.

With the guidelines, your goal will be to work up to a total of 30 minutes of cardiovascular activity per workout session. You may use a combination of the exercises listed. I suggest that beginners should start with brisk walking or jogging—whatever activity you are most comfortable with.

Core

Plank: The plank is a classic core exercise that focuses on the stability and strength of the muscles in the abdominal and surrounding areas. Engage your buttocks, press your forearms into the ground, and hold for 60 seconds. Beginners may start with a 15- to 30-second hold and work their way up.

Side plank: Another core classic and a plank variation that focuses more on the oblique muscles on either side of your central abdominals. Keep the buttocks tight and prevent your torso from sagging to get the most out of this exercise.

Woodchopper: A slightly more dynamic movement that works the rotational functionality of your core and mimics chopping a log of wood. You can start with little to no weight until you feel comfortable and progress from there. Start the move with feet shoulder-width apart, back straight, and slightly crouched. If you are using weight, hold it with both hands next to the outside of either thigh, twist to the side, and lift the weight across and upward, keeping your arms straight and turning your torso such that you end up with the weight above your opposite shoulder.

Lower Body

Goblet squat: Start your stance with feet slightly wider than shoulder width and a dumbbell held tightly with both hands in front of your chest. Sit back into a squat, hinging at both the knee and the hip joint, and lower your legs until they are parallel to the ground. Push up through your heels to the starting position and repeat. Use a chair to squat onto if you don't feel comfortable.

Dumbbell walking lunge: Start upright with a dumbbell in each hand and feet in your usual standing position. Step forward with one leg and sink until your back knee is just above the ground. Remain upright and ensure the front knee does not bend over the toes. Push through the heel of the front foot and step forward and through with your rear foot. Start with no weights, and add weight as you feel comfortable.

Upper Body

Push-ups: These are the ultimate body-weight exercise and can be done just about anywhere. You will want to set up with your hands just beyond shoulder width, keeping your body in a straight line and always engaging your core as you ascend and descend, without letting your elbows flare out. Those who struggle to perform push-ups consecutively can start by performing them on their knees or even against a wall if regular push-ups sound like too much.

Dumbbell shoulder press: An excellent exercise for upper-body and shoulder strength. Bring a pair of dumbbells to ear level, palms forward, and straighten your arms overhead.

Full Body

Mountain climbers: On your hands and feet, keep your body in a straight line, with your abdominal and buttocks muscles engaged, similar to the top position of a push-up. Rapidly alternate pulling your knees into your chest while keeping your core tight. Continue in this left, right, left, right rhythm as if you are replicating a running motion. Always try to keep your spine in a straight line.

Push press: This is essentially a combination move incorporating a partial squat and a dumbbell shoulder press. Using a weight that you are comfortable with, stand feet slightly beyond shoulder width, with light dumbbells held in a pressing position. Descend for a squat to a depth you feel comfortable with, and on the ascent simultaneously push the dumbbells overhead.

Burpee (advanced/optional): This is a classic full-body exercise that is essentially a dynamic combination of a push-up, a squat, and a jump. This particular exercise is beneficial but may be challenging for some and should be utilized only by those who feel comfortable. The proper sequencing of the movement involves starting from a standing position before lowering into a squat, placing your hands on the floor, and land on the balls of your feet while keeping your core healthy. Jump back to your hands and jump again into the air, reaching your hands upward.

Chapter 18

Law of Attraction – The Foundation of Everything you bring into your Life

Most people don't have any idea what the law of attraction is. Because it has become so popular lately, most people make it seem like a simple, magical process where you just imagine the things you want and then miraculously it appears in front of you. This process is so not really about how the law of attraction works.

This universal law is a lot more complicated than what everyone makes it out to be. The sad thing about these false facts is that they cause people to say the law of attraction doesn't work at all just because it didn't give them what they wanted.

The law of attraction does work. There is no way that it can fail. This is the way the universe has and is going to work for all eternity. Law of Attraction is a lot like the Law of Gravity. You won't ever see it, and you aren't even aware it is there. If you watch closely, you can see it in action.

Knowing how to use the law of attraction will take some time. It is a skill that needs to be cultivated but manifesting it is going to take some time. Patience is the best quality you can have during this time. I am going to try my best to explain it in a way that you will be able to understand but comprehensive enough that you will be able to use it. The first thing you need to understand is another law of the universe, and this is the law of attraction. Everything from the most significant planets and stars that live in outer space to the smallest grain of sand on the beaches will continuously be vibrating.

This is hard to believe since everything around us looks and feels solid. If everything is vibrating, why can't we put our hands through a brick wall? The answer can be found in terms of arrangement and frequency.

Our brains are so smart that it takes all the vibrations that are around us and figured out a way to make it our reality in ways that we won't ever see its waves. Think about this and look around you right now, what colours do you see? If you have taken a science class, then you know colours are another vibration that vibrates at a particular frequency. What sounds do you hear right now? They aren't anything more than a vibration that our brains have translated just to make sense from it.

If you can understand all this, you can say that your whole reality is in your head. There isn't anything out there even though we think there is. It is the same as the old question: "If a tree falls in the woods and nobody's there to hear it, does it make a sound?" The thought that you can't experience reality without actually perceiving it is the basis of the law of attraction.

Once you know that everything is vibrating, it is still hard to grasp this emotionally. This shows you that our logic is weak when compared to emotions. Logically accepting this is a lot different than believing this truth and then being able to use it in your life.

Hang in there; it will make sense in a little bit.

For you to start to create your reality on a conscious level, begin believing that everything is made up of vibrations. Take a few minutes from your day and just sit still. Try to see the vibrations of nature. Get your mind quiet and feel all the vibrations in the air around you. Get rid of any doubts that you might have for a short time and just try. You might be amazed.

Like Will Attract Like

The next thing you need to understand about the law of vibration is that similar frequencies are drawn together.

Think about two drops of water that are moving toward one another very slowly. What do you think is going to happen when they get closer? Once they get close enough to each other, they are going to attract each other and form one water drop rather than staying as two separate ones. This happens because they are of the same vibration. Think about this again but use one drop of water and a drop of oil. It doesn't matter how close you put them, and they won't ever become one. This is because they have different vibrations and are just too different.

This is the whole idea that the law of attractions is based on. If you would like to bring something into your life, and it doesn't matter what it is, start vibrating at its level.

Think About It

If everything vibrates and vibrations of same frequencies get drawn together, and you can control your vibrations. You will be able to manage your life.

The problem is going to happen when we try to control our reality without adjusting our vibrations. It won't matter how much you try to manipulate your world, and it isn't going to make the world that you want to see. The work we need to do is in our minds. This is saying that it isn't going to matter how much action we put toward something, we won't ever get the results we want. But when you can get the ability to change our minds to the desired frequency, our physical reality will soon follow suit. It will reflect this new vibration for us.

Take some time to think about all of this and see if it makes sense to you both emotionally and logically. If you believe hard enough, you might come up with the same conclusions that humanity's great leaders have come to, and that is everyone creates their reality.

Success, Money, Relationships, and Joy

The law of attraction is working at this very moment in time for your life. You are always in a creative state. You create your reality each moment of each day. You create your future with each thought, whether it is done subconsciously or consciously. There isn't any way to get away from it, and you can't ever decide not to create since it doesn't stop.

Knowing how the law of attraction works in your life is the primary key to your success. If you need or want to change your life, and you would like to empower yourself so you can have a great future, then you have to know your role in the law of attraction.

Expect Miracles

The law of attraction can provide you with infinite joy, abundance, possibilities. It doesn't understand the difficulty, and it could change your life in every possible way.

For you to know exactly how the law of attraction works, you have to look at some things.

To make it simple, the law of attraction states that you are going to attract all the things you focus on. The items you give your attention and energy to is going to come back to you.

If you remain focused on positive and good things, you will begin to attract more positive and good deeds. If you only focus on negative and bad things, this is what you will attract to your life.

Let's break it down more:

If like will attract like this means if you are feeling abundant, appreciative, joyful, happy, passionate, enthusiastic, or excited, then you will be sending out a lot of positive energy.

But if you feel sad, resentful, angry, stressed, anxious, or bored, you will be sending out negative energy.

The universe uses the law of attraction to respond to these vibrations. The universe won't decide which one is best for you, and it only responds to the energy you are sending out, and it will give you the same in return. You will get back everything you put out.

Whatever you feel and think at any time is your request for the universe to give you more of it. Since your vibrations are going to attract the same vibrations back to you, you have to be sure that you are continually sending out feelings, thoughts, and energy that resonate with the things you want to experience, do, and be.

Your energy vibrations have to be in tune with the things you want to bring into your life.

If love and joy are the things you want to attract, then the vibrations of love and happiness are the things you want to create.

Chapter 19
The Truth about the Law of Attraction that Nobody Ever Told You

Take a quick moment right now, close your eyes, and for the next ten seconds take a few deep easy breaths picturing yourself on a beach holding hands with someone you're deeply in love with.

That moment you experienced (along with the thoughts behind it) literally just shot out and instantly touched the furthest reaches of the universe. This is no exaggeration.

It's a bit like when you're on a phone call with someone on a completely different continent. Your phone transmits the signal of your voice through satellite towers, and the person on the other end hears what you say to them INSTANTLY.

That's how fast the visualization of you on the beach from a minute ago transmitted across the galaxy. Think of the enormity of this! You may not consciously notice it happening, but it IS happening.

It's like a dog whistle. You never hear any sound coming out of it, but every canine around you reacts. So it must be there. It's just on a frequency of vibration that your senses aren't designed to detect or interpret in your reality. This is SO important, and if you could perceive everything that's truly going on around you, you'd probably go insane from sensory overload.

And not just "tangible" things like the sound from a dog whistle. "Intangible" energies of the universe (many of which match the frequency of the things you want) are also literally swirling together right now -- JUST outside the boundaries of physical reality (and your physical senses) -- ready to materialize the moment, there's enough momentum.

You can't see and feel them again. You aren't experiencing them yet. But they're there. Or should I say - they're HERE? With you. Right now. They're all vibrationally where you are the MOMENT you "ask" for them (i.e. think about them).

And each one begins sending out a 'beacon' the second you "ask" -- persistently reaching out to magnetize itself to anything that vibrationally matches the same frequency.

You wouldn't be entirely wrong if you viewed these "thoughts" as conscious beings in their own right whose mission in life is finding something that matches their vibration in your time and space reality so that they can "stick" to it and physically manifest.

You're going to use the techniques in this book to match the signals of those things that you want. And in case you're feeling a bit intimidated and are wondering how you're going to do this, remember -- it's way more straightforward than you think it is. The act of doing the techniques themselves will handle everything for you without you having to make it happen consciously.

You're a bit like a radio in this way. You can only broadcast one station at a time, but you have access to every station out there.

And once you're on the station that you need to be, the music plays all by itself for you.

Now when we're talking about an ACTUAL radio, it's merely about placing your hand on the dial and turning it to the other frequencies. But when it comes to manifesting what you want through the Law of Attraction, shifting to the frequency of what you want is technically easy and straightforward.

You only think it's difficult because you're not used to doing it yet. So you worry that you don't know HOW to do it, and you then wrongly assume it can't be done for you.

But rest assured that the dial on your radio can always be turned. All you have to worry about is deciding where to put your focus (which the techniques will take care of for you) AND remember that your point of power is always NOW.

Everything You Want Is Happening Right Now!

Have you ever noticed how time can seem to go fast when you're enjoying yourself or slow when you're miserable?

This idea may seem a bit 'out there' and tough to grasp, but ask yourself how you think you'd react to being told the earth is round if you had spent your entire life up until now believing it was flat.

Are you able to hop into a space shuttle right now and prove the answer one way or another? Do you have the money, the willingness, or even the military clearance to do that? ...OR do you just have to take it on faith and trust that this is how it is?

You've got to be willing to see things in a new way without panicking.

This notion that everything is happening 'now' is important because your consciousness is rearranging subatomic particles (which determine what you experience in your time and space reality) based on your vibrational set point. And your set point is determined by your focus. And you can only control what you focus on NOW in the present moment.

In other words, your power to change your life and create your reality is always (and only) "NOW." You're not "hopefully" creating your future – it's already here! It's just a matter of needing to tune in to the right frequency to have the experience of it. But whether you're tuned in or not, it's still all here happening right now.

If this isn't entirely clear for any reason, don't worry -- it doesn't need to be clear for the techniques in this book to work. And the instructions for them will be very simple to use. Just know that you have access to a lot more power than you'll ever realize. Technically, on a certain level, you have access to EVERYTHING.

Because everything is energy, including you, and here's an important little fact about the energy that you may not have considered before now.

Energy cannot be created or destroyed.

All you can do at any moment is transform it.

But it's all here, and it always will be. Which means,

Everything that could EVER exist already DOES ...in this present moment of NOW.

It may not currently be in the manifested form of that car you've wanted...or the love of your life or the promotion you've been going after -- but it still all energetically exists. It's still all "here" waiting for you in the potential, ready to be pulled into reality through your point of attraction. And that means,

Everything you also want ALREADY exists!

Every desire you've ever had already exists RIGHT NOW. This isn't some wacky claim. This is SCIENCE. This is the LAW. And experiencing what you want simply then becomes a question of using the right techniques to line up with it and manifest it energetically. Simple as that. But it's all still just an energy construct.

Thoughts are an energy construct.

"Time" is an energy construct.

Money is an energy construct.

Reality is an energy construct.

EVERYTHING is an energy construct.

Your raise at work, your car, your new boyfriend or girlfriend, your new book deal, your original contract, your new apartment, your new house, your improved health -- it's all just energy. And it's all connected. Your whole life, you've been conditioned to believe that everything you want is "out there" ...somewhere else ...at another point in time.

And ironically, it's your belief in this "separation" from what you want that reinforces the reality that you don't have it yet. This includes your certainty in the concept of time and getting what you want "in the future" vs. already having it "now." That's why things seem so much harder to get than they should. But there's no such thing as "now" and "later" to the universe. And there's no such thing as "big" and "small."

Unfortunately, you've been programmed for so long to see a distinction between "big" and "small" that hearing this information may sound silly or foolish to you. Especially the idea that time isn't really what you think it is.

But again, if any of this is a bit challenging, that's okay. The techniques are still the answer. They don't need you to get this right away. They don't even require you to grasp this ever. The universe is so abundant, and the techniques are so powerful that you can still have everything you want. If you realized how heavily the odds are already stacked in your favor, your head would spin.

You Are Swimming In Abundance.

It's all around you!

Right now, at THIS moment, the universe is moving through every person and every circumstance to give to you. That's all it wants to do. Countless things are already going well for you, whether you see them or not. Even in moments of struggle, the universe is holding you up and keeping solutions just close enough for you to reach out and claim them.

Do you ever have to worry if the sun will come up? Do you ever wonder if the earth will continue to spin? Do you ever need to worry that you're going to run out of air or water? Of course not, but how much harder would your life be if you had to worry about these kinds of things?

Fortunately, you don't have to worry, and just as your heartbeat is already being taken care of for you, so is that job offer you want that's way closer than you think (and just waiting for you to adjust your radio dial a TINY bit). Remember, this is the same universe that created this planet, the entire solar system, and every star in existence, the birds that sing every morning, the cool breeze on a warm beach, and the love of your life, your favorite song, and everything else! There's a vibrational version of your love, your money, your new house, your new car, your health, your prosperity, your success, and anything else you could ever want that exists RIGHT NOW. It's all here, right at your fingertips!

Which begs the question, if you're swimming in an energetic pool of abundance if everything you've ever desired wants you just as much if there are infinite resources at your disposal if the universe loves you and desperately desires to offer you anything and everything you could ever think of…Why hasn't anything worked out yet? Why hasn't the Law of

Attraction given you what you want? Why are you still struggling? What's going on here? What are you missing?

These questions all have the very same (and simple) answer.

And once you understand what has been holding you back, it will never have any power over you ever again.

Chapter 20
Stop Emotional Eating

We don't know we're an emotional eater for most of us, or we don't think it's that severe. For some of us, it doesn't lead to feelings of shame or weight gain. We can console some of us and think it's not a big deal, but it's not.

Among others, emotional eating is out of balance, something that can dominate our everyday lives. This may seem like overwhelming cravings or hunger, but it's just the feeling that we feel hungry, helpless and add to our weight.

Comfort food gives us immediate pleasure and takes away feeling. Digestion and sensation require a lot of time, and the body can't do it. Comfort eating helps us to suppress pain because we flood our digestive tract with poisonous waste.

When we feel anxious, feeling a big empty hole inside us like we're hungry can be natural. Instead of confronting what this means — i.e. our emotions— we're stuffing it down. In culture, it seems we are afraid to feel too much that we don't even know we're running from our feelings much of the time.

If we don't let ourselves react, we'll repress it. You will feel exhausted until you begin to let yourself feel the thoughts or feelings that emerge and avoid stuffing down. It is because the body releases past pent-up emotions, and it can strike you hard.

That's why it can be hard to let go of emotional eating, as we have to conquer the initial "scare" to move on and start learning to accept emotions for what they are. To be present, allowing a feeling to wash over us is wonderful and should be appreciated.

The more you allow yourself to be in the present moment and feel, the fewer feelings that overtake you, the less terrified you will be. The emotion's strength also decreases. You'll become mentally and physically stronger. When it's off your stomach, you'll feel so much better than replacing it with food.

Getting to this point isn't fast. Some people can split their emotional eating by better nourishing their body to get rid of physical cravings and supporting others when they feel anxious or emotional.

To stop emotional eating, you must be mindful of how and why you eat—taking a day out to consider what makes you happy. Many people don't even understand real hunger!

When you're eating mentally, can you stop yourself?

Could you sit and let the emotion wash over you instead of eating-give yourself time to feel it and transfer it? Or would you talk to someone about how you feel?

Don't injure yourself.

Emotional eating is usually something you've done from an early age because it's part of your make-up. It's a practised habit, so you've learned to cope with the environment.

It takes time to undo something so ingrained in you, so if you find yourself eating out of guilt-if, you mess up-learn from it, just move on. Recognition is the first step. If you know you eat safely, you can conquer it.

Journaling will also help you recognize eating habits. Note down before, during and after a meal. What caused eating-was real hunger?

To learn how to avoid emotional eating, I can help. For years, I suffered from an emotional eating epidemic, sometimes going on a day-to-day binge eating marathon. I never really understood what caused these eating outbursts, all I knew was that I would start eating and not stop until the food was gone, or anyone near me saw me.

The situation escalated, and my weight started to increase. Any diet I was on would instantly fail, and my self-confidence reached an all-time low. My eating causes were thought to be related to work stress, but so many others may play a part. Relationships, depression, financial difficulties, and many others will easily consume binge sequence.

When I started trying to figure out how to avoid emotional eating, I didn't know where to start. Like you, I went online and started investigating. I spent the whole day reading, digesting, and gathering emotional cure knowledge, then around 3 a.m. I found my savior that morning.

And how can you avoid emotional eating?

The answer is very easy. The trick is identifying the real root cause of the problems and addressing those root causes. You may think its tension or job issues. Yet mental eating disorders are also much more profound than on the surface. Following the root, a cause can quickly treat these symptoms and safely cure your binge eating.

Mental eating satisfies your mental appetite. It's not about your kitchen, but the issue lies in your head. What are the most powerful emotional eating challenge strategies?

List your food cravings to relax.

Distracting yourself doesn't mean being lazy in this situation. It's not like texting while driving, or you're out of control. When you hide from your food cravings, it means you're turning your focus to something else. It's more purposeful.

Do something or concentrate on another action or event. Whenever you feel like gorging food, try getting a piece of paper and list five items from five categories of something like the names of five people whenever you feel upset, angry or depressed.

Perhaps you should mention five ways to relax. If you want to calm down, what are your five places?

When anxious, what five feel-good phrases can you tell yourself? How about five things to stop eating?

Place on your fridge or kitchen cabinet after finishing this list. Next time you're overwhelmed by your persuasive food cravings, browse through your list and do one of the 25 things suggested there.

Prepare ahead for future emotional issues.

Over the weekend, grab a piece of paper and a pencil and take a path to your tasks in the days ahead. Your map reveals your expected exits and potential detours. Pick an emotionally consuming picture.

Place the icon over an event or activity that could cause your food cravings, like early lunch with your in-laws. Prepare ahead for that case. Search for the restaurant menu online to order something delicious and nutritious.

Drop the concerns inside.

Whenever anxious, taking a deep breath helps. Another thing to detoxify yourself from stress is to do a visual trick. Breathe deeply and imagine a squeegee (that piece of cloth you use to clean your window or windshield) near your eyes. Slowly breathe out, picture the squeegee wiping clean inside. Delete all your concerns. Do it three times.

Self-talk like you're royalty. Self-criticism is usually emotional. Toxic words you say to yourself, such as "I'm such a loser" or "I can never seem to do anything right," force you to drive to the nearest. Don't be fooled by these claims though brief.

Such feelings, like acid rain, slowly erode your well-being. The next time you're caught telling yourself these negative things, overcome by moving to a third-person perspective.

If you think "I'm such a mess," tell yourself then that "Janice is such a mess, but Janice will do what it takes to get things done and make herself happy."

This approach will get you out of the negative self-talk loop and have some perspective. Pull up and be positive and have the strength and avoid emotional eating.

Over-food is still not given enough consideration. It's always seen as not a serious problem to laugh at.

This is an incorrect view as a horrific condition needing urgent treatment. The positive thing is that you take action to help you avoid emotional eating forever. I know because I did it myself.

Step1-Recognize triggers

For each person, emotional eating is triggered differently. Some people get cravings when stressed out, some when depressed or bored. You need to try and work out the emotional causes. When you know what they are, you'll get an early notice when the urge to feed comes on you.

Step 2-Eliminate Temptation

One thing most people don't realize about emotional eating is that desire is always for one specific food. It's always ice-cream or candy for kids. It's still pizza for guys.

When you couldn't fulfil this lure, it won't bother you. Save your home from all of these temptations.

Throw out any nearby pizza delivery locations. Again, you know your tempters, so get rid of them and make overeating difficult.

Step 3-Break contact

It's instant and urgent when craving hits. You're fed RIGHT NOW! To stop this, you must break this immediate bond by taking some time between desires and eating.

Call a friend Count to 60

Write down what you feel like

Do some exercises go out for a walk

Take a shower

What you can do to make the urge subside do wonder.

Take these three moves, and you'll soon take them better and conquer emotional eating for good.

Chapter 21

Habits for Weight Loss Success

Understanding Habit

If you try to make a difference in your life, you're working to alter old habits and to create new ones. Sitting down and thinking about the improvements you want in your life is easy, but they are hard to execute and keep going. It's because you've produced patterns that need to be changed to be successful.

I have taught a lot of customers in my career, and almost every customer I teach knows what they have to do to achieve their target, but they can't. How do you do that?

Since they don't choose to take the necessary action periodically to develop habits that will produce long-term results.

Our customs control our actions. Understanding habits and their role in your life is essential, as they are responsible for your daytime choices. An individual does not lose weight because he or she is not aware that during commercial breaks, he or she is used to going to the kitchen to eat. For some instances, habit is something we don't know about. We do so consciously. Being mindful of your habits gives you the strength to make your life-changing decision. It's hard to make a decision when you know what your options are.

It's essential to be mindful of your old habits and the new ones you need to create while you are making changes in your life. Just think about the change you'd like to make. (Lose weight, get in shape, and get more energy) Now think about where you are right now, and what shift you want to make. (Lose 30 lbs., have more stamina, build strength, have more energy) Now think about the past and the acts you've taken, which are responsible for where you're at. (Eat fast food, watch TV, and drink too much, every night).

Now ask yourself what actions do I need to take to bring about the change that I want to see in my life? The solutions you'll come up with are the acts you need to turn into behaviors. A habit is something you do, and you do not worry about it. You need to do the behavior regularly to build this habit before you have to think about it.

Habits aren't instantly created. It's something you have to do, consistently, for an extended period. How long does it take to do this? When you do it, and you do not have to worry about it. I read a lot of different stuff about how long it takes to build a habit ... Thirty days, sixty, ninety days ... I think these are fantastic goals, but I know it may take you a little longer. If this is a move that you want to make, you're going to do the research and work hard to make it happen.

Habits can be divided into two categories: motor and (actually) mental habits.

We reflect daily ways of acting or thinking we know without grappling with our will or even voluntary strength. Habits are acquired by learning, and then particularly by repetition.

It is, therefore, essential that the components (acts or thoughts) be replicated regularly and several times until a new habit is created.

Running, walking, walking, driving and so on are things that we had to know.

When we understand habits, we usually think of the behavior we replicate, and the habit of science will tell us why we replicate our patterns and develop habits as we grow up.

Habits are also repeated patterns of actions and behaviors that we are conditioned to perform, and that can evolve over many years, and habits that have evolved over many years are more likely to be stronger than those that have been developed recently or in a few years.

And habits that we learn as children remain with us all our lives are more likely than habits that we learn as adults. And the frequency or success of those habits would be directly linked to how long we have had those patterns of behavior.

And this is the routine that we all formed as children waking up in the morning and brushing our teeth. Now we have to wonder what if we're trying to stop the habits? What if we wake up, and have not brushed our teeth? Besides the fact that we can end up with bad breath when we don't obey one of our everyday routines, there are real psychological effects of physical and emotional or social distress!

Brushing your teeth is a case in point. Another could be when you enter your apartment and turn on the TV or computer shortly after you return home. In your immediate area, you immediately feel uncomfortable if you stop doing so, even if it's your own home, as though something is missing from your life.

Suppose your TV or laptop is broken down, you can't exercise the habit, and you feel depressed. We, humans, are slaves to these patterns of behavior, and thus habits are an important part of our lives. This discomfort we feel can be seen as the product of 'habit obstruction' when we are unable to exercise our habits. Thus the effects of disruption of habit may have a significant effect on our emotional, social and personal lives.

If habit obstruction effect is long-term, that is when your laptop is broken for weeks or months. You can't turn it on when you enter your house or apartment, and the habit obstruction effect will spread to habit hunger. After a few weeks of habit obstruction, you may even start losing your habit subconsciously when you get into the habit hunger effect.

So habit hunger can cause some form of amnesia from your usual behavior, and you forget about that habit. It's all very good, but then not so simple, because you might have some form of habit displacement in this case and develop some other habit.

The Importance of Habits

Behind every habit, there is a real need that you need to satisfy. Be it any kind of habit, good or bad. Like for example:

- Who smokes to relieve stress?

- Who drinks to relax?
- Whoever exercises for pleasure?

All of these activities, whether harmful or not, contain a yearning for fulfilment for those who practice. This is what makes a habit so challenging to change.

So much so that when trying to change a habit, you will experience great difficulty in the first few weeks.

Because, when you stop doing something that was already customary, your body will begin to crave that sensation caused by that old custom that you left behind.

Tips to improve your habits

Life is full of habits, good and bad, it is just as easy to have positive habits as negative, but transforming them implies an effort and a lot of willpower, a change of beliefs and appreciation.

The answer is in you, can you change your habits?

- Know the habits you would like to adopt. Start by making a detailed list of the habits you would like to change or improve.
- Analyze the attitudes that general conflicts. If you have not been able to identify all the bad habits or do not think you do not have them, ask yourself what kind of behaviors generate conflicts in your daily life and with the people around you, an example would be if you arrive at your appointments late and this causes discomfort in other people if you

have no energy because you do not eat healthily or if you are a little overweight and you dislike it.

· Become aware of the importance of changing bad habits. It is important to raise awareness subtly, to the people closest to you about the importance of improving their habits. If they do it simultaneously, it will be easier to adopt them. For example, if someone in your family buys junk food and you are looking for a healthy diet, it is vital to encourage them not to do so that everyone improves their habits and their diet, especially if this person is overweight.

· Build an action plan. Once you have identified the habits you would like to adopt, you need to make an action plan to carry it out. The first step is to become aware of the habit you want to change and continuously monitor your actions and thinking patterns to identify why you react that way. The next thing will be to repeat the new habit every day for at least 30 days, and it is the minimum time in which a habit is adopted. For example, if you want to start exercising, do it at least four days a week for two months. In this way, your body and mind will adapt to the new activities you do.

· Be honest with yourself. Finally, you must be objective and recognize if you have continued repeating the new habits, analyze if you already feel that they are part of your daily life. If not, it is important to examine the causes that prevented you from achieving it.

Habits are nothing more than the daily repetition of an attitude and discipline. The best day to start changing your habits is today. If you stop to think about all the time it takes to change a habit, and you probably won't, the important thing is to be determined and start today.

How to Improve Your Eating Habits For Weight Loss

The barriers people have reached for themselves seem to have no end in sight. Hunger, fruit diets and uncooked foods are among the drastic alternatives to the long old weight-loss problem. I had attempted to try these for myself, and none of them succeeded until I closed the diet and only changed my weight loss eating habits.

The diets are similar to weight loss band-aids. In a short-term illness, they are a fast solution and do not change behavior, metabolism or produce a true bang on body fat. Dietary rigidity does not increase the element of success; in reality, it decreases it. It is much easier to make gradual changes that are not upsetting or penalizing but launch the body on the road to equilibrium and its normal set point to some extent. Stable changes in eating habits are certainly an excellent option for losing weight.

Rather than eliminating calories by the end of the day or for a big meal, five or six small food portions are much healthier for the body. This sounds contradictory but real. The body burns calories in everyday exercise. This requires food calories to feed and digest. Reports show that up to 10% of calories are used to process the food.

Therefore, 50 calories are needed for food processing for a 500-calorie serving. It's been shown that eating less often helps in weight gain over the long term. To strengthen your weight-loss eating habits, you will regularly consume yet healthy foods. A psychosomatic eating benefit is feeling good. The feeling you're not hollow is beneficial in continuing the weight loss cycle.

Booming weight loss isn't a major science, nor does it entail difficulty and pain—easy changes like cooking nutritious meals 5-6 times a day. Eating the right part size is critical. Eating the right calories is important, and daily exercise is important. Eat and consume the right form of food are the safest dietary habits for weight loss.

Chapter 22
Hypnosis Myths

It is common to misjudge the topic of hypnotism. That is why myths and half-truths abound about this matter.

Myth: You won't recall that anything that happened when you were mesmerized when you wake up from a trance.

While amnesia may occur in uncommon cases, during mesmerizing, people more often than not recollect everything that unfolded. Mesmerizing, be that as it may, can have a significant memory impact. Posthypnotic amnesia may make an individual overlook a portion of the stuff that occurred previously or during spellbinding. This effect, be that as it may, is typically confined and impermanent.

Myth: Hypnosis can help people to recall the exact date of wrongdoing they have been seeing.

While spellbinding can be utilized to improve memory, the effects in well-known media have been significantly misrepresented. Research has discovered that trance doesn't bring about noteworthy memory improvement or precision, and entrancing may, in reality, lead to false or misshaped recollections.

Myth: You can be spellbound against your will

Spellbinding needs willful patient investment regardless of stories about people being mesmerized without their authorization.

Myth: While you are under a trance, the trance specialist has full power over your conduct.

While individuals frequently feel that their activities under trance appear to happen without their will's impact, a trance specialist can't make you act against your wants.

Myth: You might be super-solid, brisk, or physically gifted with trance.

While mesmerizing can be utilized for execution upgrade, it can't make people more grounded or more athletic than their physical abilities.

Myth: Everyone can be entranced

It is beyond the realm of imagination to expect to entrance everybody. One research shows that it is amazingly hypnotizable around 10 percent of the populace. While it might be attainable to spellbind the rest of the masses, they are more reluctant to be open to the activity.

Myth: You are responsible for your body during trance

Despite what you see with stage trance, you will remain aware of what you are doing and what you are being mentioned. On the off chance that you would prefer not to do anything under mesmerizing, you're not going to do it.

Myth: Hypnosis is equivalent to rest.

You may look like resting, yet during mesmerizing, you are alert. You're just in a condition of profound unwinding. Your muscles will get limp, your breathing rate will back off, and you may get sleepy.

Myth: When mesmerized, individuals can't lie,

Sleep induction isn't a truth serum in the real world. Even though during subliminal therapy, you are progressively open to a recommendation, regardless, you have through and through freedom and good judgment. Nobody can make you state anything you would prefer not to say — lie or not.

Myth: Many cell phone applications and web recordings empower self-trance, yet they are likely inadequate.

Analysts in a 2013 survey found that such instruments are not ordinarily created by an authorized trance inducer or mesmerizing association. Specialists and subliminal specialists consequently prescribe against utilizing these.

Most likely, a myth: entrancing can help you "find" lost recollections.

Even though recollections can be recouped during mesmerizing, while in a daze like a state, you might be bound to create false recollections, along these lines, numerous trance specialists remain distrustful about memory recovery utilizing spellbinding.

The primary concern entrancing holds the stage execution generalizations, alongside clacking chickens and influential artists.

Trance, be that as it may, is a genuine remedial instrument and can be utilized for a few conditions as elective restorative treatment. This includes the administration of a sleeping disorder, grief, and agony.

You utilize a trance specialist or subliminal specialist authorized to confide in the technique for guided trance. An organized arrangement will be made to help you accomplish your individual goals.

Chapter 23
Weight Control Individualization

Individualization of a particular program is being stressed, and more of this is still going to happen. If you want the plan you choose to work with to be most effective and produce beautiful results, you must make it yours and ensure that it is unique to you according to what you think can work well for you. Do not start using a program that is not individualized, one that you pick from anywhere and start using because it may not work for you. As you already know, as an individual, you have a unique retinal pattern, fingerprints, and the body chemistry you have does not match that of anyone else. The things you have experienced in life are also different from those of other people.

In the same way, a program that you can use to help you in attaining a unique bodyweight should also be unique to you so that it can achieve maximum positive results. This is why you can see that here you are only provided with a few meditation exercises that you have the chance to choose the best ones that suits you. Giving you so many meditation exercises may be overwhelming when it comes to choosing the activity that suits your body and the one that you are comfortable with. When you are overwhelmed with many choices of meditation exercises to choose from, there is the possibility that you may be confused about making the right decision. Also, you can see that no meditation has been given in a stone manner, the only part that you need to put a lot of effort to ensure success is maintaining your discipline and telling yourself that you know the kind of goals you want. It would be best if you achieved them no matter what happens as you proceed with these exercises.

As an individual, you should discover which form suits you best and follow that diligently until you get the results that you aim for. Many people all over the world have tried meditation methods. Still, many of them have failed because most teachers for meditational schools believe that there is one way to meditate, which applies to each and every one throughout the world. Many think that they have learned this method from their meditation schools and their teacher through coincidence and by being curious. But the truth is that this could be their best meditation method as individuals, but it does not mean everyone else will find it comfortable, and by using it, they must achieve success. Such kinds of people who have been disappointed because they did not get the results they expected from the meditation exercises belief that it cannot work for them, yet they have not tried other forms of meditation and see how it can work for them.

However, particular aspects come in all forms of meditational paths. For example, meditators should try to continually arrive at the maximum attention possible, which is called coherent attention in some meditational schools. This is whereby, as an individual, you decide to discipline your mind and ensure always to do one thing at a particular time to maintain focus and avoid being overwhelmed. You also decide that you love yourself, and you will treat yourself in a manner that you have promised yourself. These are some of the constants when it comes to various meditational schools. Apart from these, the other things that are involved like doing your meditation while walking in the area of your comfort, do it while sitting in an armchair, and lying on the floor are things that you should decide for yourself and consider the one that you are comfortable with. When it comes to deciding the best time for you to perform the meditational exercises; it is up to you, and there is no conventional way in which you should follow. You can choose to be doing it either once or twice in a day and perform them for one, two, or three weeks depending on what you have promised yourself that you will achieve.

As you continue, if you find that you are committed, and you have a great desire to achieve the healthy body weight that you need to have, you can decide to follow all the meditational exercises because overall, they will help you to achieve your goals. If you do not want to try different meditational paths, then you can decide to go for the combined meditations that you have explicitly identified. There are various forms of meditations that you can choose to go with. Some of these meditational paths include those that stress on the intellectual path, that those enable you to work through emotions and others that have been devised by religious groups in the western world. It does not matter the form of meditation that you have decided to use to attain your goals and experience fulfilment. The truth is that to achieve what you want with these various kinds of meditations. You must put in the work that is required. The results will not be easy for any form of meditation that you decide to go with. Be sure that whatever path you choose, you will not find any easy path because achieving the growth and development you want is difficult. The only best way to achieve what you want is that you be serious and be prepared to put an effort that will not stop soon.

These statements may seem to be put strongly, but those who have attempted to change their lives and succeeded can attest to this and tell you that it is the truth. When we work to achieve a healthy body weight through meditation, we need to know that we will not only individualize our meditational programs but also there are other aspects of our lives that we should also individualize. We will look at some of these things that we should put into considering when it comes to individualizing the program we have.

For many years, individualization has not been taken seriously, and many have underrated it. Even some experienced psychiatrists do not seem to get it, and many of them may not understand that various patients need different help when it comes to psychotherapy. These people also need various preparedness measures to deal with impending stress due to surgery, and they should be helped differently so that they can effectively deal with allergies, grief, and other issues affecting their lives. But the modern concept does not need to incorporate this hence the reason you see why many meditations have been conditioned to think that there is a particular method of performing psychotherapy that is correct and can be used on various patients and this is the method that they learned from their teachers and mastered it carefully.

Those who try to come up with different concepts both meditation teachers and patients do not succeed in convincing others that there is a need for an individualized program for everyone for it to work well and for the patient to succeed. Many find it easy to believe that there is only one way regardless of what you are dealing with, whether it is meditation, psychotherapy, or other things that need treatment.

They do not want to face the complex situation that every one of different and the best way is to deal with each individual differently, whether this is something complicated or not. However, it would help if you got that we are different individuals with different bodies. When thinking of exercises, do not go for what has been hyped but design your individualized program because this is what can help you get the best results and follow your journey to becoming what you want to become. Are you thinking of changing the movement exercise that you have been doing? If you do not have such an exercise you are doing currently, you can add in your daily program. By looking around, try to know what is appealing to you. You can find an exercise that you are happy with. The kind of exercise you choose should be one that after you are through with the performance, you are left feeling good. If you are good with the popular exercise at the moment, you can go for it, and this could be a sweet coincidence. As you choose the exercise, you need to consider some factors like your current age, the pattern of exercises you were engaged in, and your physique. If you are okay with it, you may decide that you combine several of these exercises and add them to the specific regimen that you already have. You may choose to be jogging every morning, swimming a few laps on two days of the week, and taking a walk on days like Sundays.

As you may have already realized, the subject of the right path for each person, lacking has been stressed in this book. Meditation is also not left out, which is one of the best ways to solve various issues for some individuals. It is excellent for many great people around the world have appreciated many people and it but remember that some people find it to be relevant and not that helpful in their lives. If, you are devoted to these meditational exercises and conscientiously perform them for a period of six to eight weeks without seeing results, do not hate yourself because meditation is not your thing. By doing it, your weight cannot become worse, but even if you do not notice the benefits that you were looking for, the advantage that will be there is that you will have undertaken something that you have not done before. At the same time, you will also have engaged your mind to know various things that maybe you did not know about yourself and your body. Even when you find that meditation may not work best when it comes to solving your weight problem, the experience is benefitting, and it will help you learn a lot.

Chapter 24

Benefits of Being Healthy to Motivate You

The process of getting that what is necessary requires you as an individual to be able to acquire some personal discipline. Before you purchase any food, you need to ask yourself if buying the food is necessary. Ask yourself if the food that you are eating will add any value to your overall health. After asking yourself that question, you will know the right thing to do based on the response to the questions. It is an easy process to do, and it will help to save you from eating those carbs that only add unnecessary weight to your body.

Maintain a healthy body

Once we consume food, our bodies respond to what we have consumed. The response could be negative or positive. Different foods generate different feelings. You may not believe what some of these feelings are, except you focus your minds on realizing them. The power of meditation is that it allows you to be able to focus, concentrate on a particular thing that requires your attention. This is an easy task to accomplish, and you only should evaluate how your body reacts to the foods that you are consuming. Once you eat some foods, you will notice that you feel energized, while some foods will make you feel tired.

Once you overeat, you will experience some sudden feelings of tiredness. You will begin to feel as if your body is too heavy, and so all you want to do is take a nap or a rest. Now when this happens, you should realize that it is a sign that whatever you ate was unnecessary, and hence the body will not use the food. As a result, most of what you ate will become something that your body needs to eliminate. Thus, you will start to add extra weight, because the excess food in your body becomes excess fat in your body. On the other hand, if once you eat, it immediately makes you feel energized; it means your body was receptive to the food that you eat.

It means that your body was able to convert much of the food into energy, and your body will well utilize each of that component present in the food. This is beneficial for the wellbeing of your body, and it can help you when losing weight and prevent you from adding unnecessary weight.

Maintain the bodyweight

A great many people don't comprehend that adding daze to your weight reduction endeavors can enable you to lose more weight and look after it. Spellbinding originates before the tallying of carb and calories by a few decades. However, this well-established technique for centering consideration presently can't seem to be held entirely onto as an effective methodology for weight reduction.

As of not long ago, the real claims of prestigious trance inducers have been bolstered by insufficient logical proof, and an excess of pie-in-the-sky responsibilities from their issue kin, stage trance specialists, have not made a difference.

Indeed, even after a powerful reanalysis of 18 sleep-inducing studies in the mid-1990s demonstrated that psychotherapy clients who appropriately self-trance lost twice as much weight as compared to the individuals who didn't (and held it off in one research two years after the part of the bargain) unless if you or somebody you know has joyfully been constrained by entrancing to buy a crisp, littler closet, it might be hard to believe that this psyche over-body procedure can enable you to take a few to get back some composure on eating.

Seeing is thinking absolutely. So, investigate yourself. To gain proficiency with a portion of the priceless exercises that trance must instruct about weight reduction, you don't need to be spellbound. The ten smaller than expected ideas that pursue contain a portion of the eating regimen modifying recommendations that my gathering and individual hypnotherapy weight the executive's clients get.

The power is inside. Trance specialists believe that you have all you should be effective. You truly needn't bother with an alternate accident diet or the ongoing suppressant of hunger. Thinning, as you do when you ride a bike, is tied in with confiding in your innate abilities. You may not recall how terrifying it was the point at which you previously endeavored to ride a bike. However, you kept on rehearsing until you had the option to ride, consequently, with no idea or exertion. Getting more fit may appear past you moreover. However, it's just about finding your balance.

You see your conviction. Individuals will, in general, do what they accept they can achieve. That is even valid for mesmerizing. Those fooled into deduction they could be entranced (for example, as the trance inducer proposed they would see red, he turned the switch on a disguised red bulb) demonstrated improved mesmerizing reaction. It is essential to hope to be made a difference. Give me a chance to propose you anticipate that your arrangement should work on weight reduction. Highlight the positive. Recommendations, for example, "Doughnuts will sicken you," negative or aversive, work for some time, however on the off chance that you need lasting change, you need to think emphatically. Specialists Herbert Spiegel and David Spiegel, a dad child hypnotherapy group, considered the most well-known valuable trance-like proposition. "I need my body to live in. I owe regard and security to my body." I elevate clients to create their very own energetic mantras. A 50-year-old mother who shed 50 pounds more rehashes day by day: "Superfluous nourishment is a weight on my body. I will shed what I needn't bother with."

It's going to come if you envision it. Like competitors who are getting ready for the challenge, you are set up for a successful truth by picturing triumph. Envisioning a smart dieting day will enable you to envision the means expected to turn into a decent eater. Is it too difficult to even think about photographing? Locate a comfortable old photograph of yourself and recall what you did another way. Envision these schedules reviving. Or, on the other hand, picture acquiring direction from a more former, more astute self later on in the wake of contacting her required weight.

Get rid of cravings. Subliminal specialists utilize the intensity of emblematic symbolism on a standard premise, welcoming subjects to put sustenance desires on fleecy white mists or inflatables in sight-seeing and send them up, up, and away. On the off chance that you can direct off your eating routine from McDonald's brilliant curves, trance inducers comprehend that a counter-image can control you back. Welcome your psyche to flip through its picture Rolodex until you develop as an indication of yearnings throwing out. Push.

There are two preferred procedures over one. A triumphant mix is entrancing and Cognitive Behavioral Treatment (CBT) with regards to getting more fit and holding it off, which patches up counterproductive thoughts and practices. Clients learning both lose twice as much weight without falling -a few, recuperate more trap of the health food nut. On the off chance that you'vc at any point kept up a sustenance journal, you've officially endeavored CBT. They monitor everything that experiences their lips for possibly 14 days before my clients learn mesmerizing. Each great trance inducer comprehends that raising cognizance is a principle move for the tyke towards suffering change.

Modify and then change. The late pioneer of spellbinding, Milton Erickson, MD, focused on you's essentialness. To improve the lose-recuperation, the lose-recuperation example of one customer, Erickson recommended that she put on weight first before losing it — an intense sell today, except if you're Charlize Theron. Simpler to swallow: Modify your craving for high calories.

Like it or not, it is the fittest for survival. No proposal is sufficiently able to supersede the nature of survival. Similarly, as we like to believe, it's the most appropriate survival, despite everything we're modified for survival in case of starvation. A valid example: a private dietary mentor needed a proposal for her dependence on a sticky bear. The advisor attempted to clarify that her body felt that her life relied upon the chewy desserts and wouldn't surrender them until she got enough calories from progressively nutritious food. No, she demanded, all that she required was a proposition when she dropped out.

Practice makes perfect. There are no washboard abs delivered by one Pilates class, and one spellbinding session can't shape your eating routine. Be that as it may, discreetly rehashing a useful suggestion 15 to 20 minutes every day can change your eating, especially when combined with moderate, regular breaths, the foundation of any program of social change.

Improved mental functioning

This practice is exceptionally similar to the old practice, only instead of merely visualizing the room you want to describe it to yourself. Imagine as though you are mentally chatting with yourself or someone else, and explain what the room looks like as you go about doing it. Say, for example, "The room has white walls, a white door, and white framing around the door. It has a green chair in the corner, a white desk on the north-facing wall, and a window that faces the East."

You want to describe this room down to the minutest detail you can recall for that room. Do not skip on details, describe everything you can recall. The idea is that you want to complete this exercise while also improving your attention and mental awareness. As you do this, you will be engaging in both visualization and verbalization, which can be helpful to those who are not entirely visually-oriented. You can also describe the details out loud if you feel that you need even more of a verbal to your practice.

If you are not someone who prefers to use movement to enter your trance-like state but would rather do so by remaining still and calm within yourself, then you can try taking advantage of visualization. Visualization is a great practice that allows you to take control of your mind's eye and "leave" your physical body by entering your mind, instead. The following visualization practice is a great way to get your mind in control and enter a trance-like state so that you can begin your self-hypnosis practice.

Get into a comfortable position and then let your eyes fall closed. Once they have, consider a room that you are used to entering. It can be any room that you know well, and that helps you feel comfortable.

Once you have considered the room, begin to visualize it. You want to place as many details into that room as possible. Consider the colours of the walls, the door frame, the door itself, and any windows that might be in that room. Consider the view you get on the outside of the window, and then visualize all of the contents of the room. All of the furniture, decorations, and other objects that fill the room should be "built" into your visualized version of this room.

Once you have done this, consider a room that you are less familiar with. Practice putting it together in the same way you did the room that you knew well.

Now, consider the differences between the two experiences. Notice how well you were able to mentally design the first room and your discrepancies in the second room. As you do, also notice how deep of a relaxation you have entered, and use that to help you relax further. Then, you can begin practicing your self-hypnosis practices.

Chapter 25

A New Self

Validation: Seek, and You Shall Find

Your new belief is extremely fragile until it gets locked into your identity or part of your construct of the world. You closed in your old limiting beliefs, ingraining them into your psychology, by validating them over and over again. In the same fashion—but consciously, this time—you can now make these new beliefs "real" to you.

Its job is to recognize and find everything within your environment that you have pre-determined to be vital to you. It begins to find everything that lines up with what you expect to see, specifically, what matches your beliefs. That's why you don't notice something—the car or purse you finally purchased, the type of house you chose to live in, a particular piece of jewelry that interests you—until it becomes somehow important to you.

All of a sudden, it's almost magically everywhere.

That's how you find what you're looking for. There was a point when building our speaking centre suite in Northern California when my wife and the designers started to drive me to every flooring company in the area. It seemed like the goal was for me to see every possible option of granite, travertine, limestone, hardwood, and carpeting. Apart from being fascinated at how many flooring companies seemed to pop up in town suddenly, I'm amazed at how I still can't drive by and not notice them. Even though it's been years, I can't help but see them in the corner of my eye when I drive by. The stores had always been there; they were just "invisible" until they became important to me.

Your new belief needs to become a top priority on your "Importance List"—the things your brain is selectively looking out for. Remember that your brain craves consistency in your interpretation of the matrix of the world. It's always making sure that it's validating your construct of beliefs. Whenever there's a discrepancy, that's a chance for growth and an opening for a new belief. Building up the much-needed evidence for your new belief will allow your brain to make this belief a reality.

Familiarity Breeds Identity

Remember that, according to the well-respected developmental biologist Bruce Lipton, up to 95% of our behavior is unconscious. You are less in control of what you do than you thought you were. Remember that our emotions pull the strings of our behavior. Look back at your day to day; how many of your decisions were made on auto-pilot? Did you brush your teeth the same way, using the same toothpaste, bought from the same store as always? Did you drink the same coffee, the same way as you always do? Did you drive the same route to get to your usual destination? When you first turned on your computer, did you visit the same favorite sites?

I'm not saying this is good or bad. I'm not passing judgment. I'm saying it's important to raise your awareness of this because you create your habits, and then your habits create you. Behavioral scientists, neuroscientists, and psychologists are in general agreement that it's the repetition of the same habitual patterns of thoughts, feelings, and behaviors that create your identity. Your past conditioned your old patterns. This is your blueprint, and it's your current wiring; it's how you do things because it's how you are. This is what makes change so hard. To leave the security and certainty of your old self can be uncomfortable and daunting.

That's when most will back out. They'll revert to what they know. They'll cave in and give up.

The solution is to stop living in the past. You can't create a different future otherwise. Change happens the moment your mind stops living in the conditioned programs of the past and starts living for the future.

Chapter 26
Psychology of Weight Loss

If you have carried on with most of your life overweight, you've in all probability attempted many weight loss programs, weight loss diets and a substantial portion of medications and pills for sure. Any individual who has experienced these encounters realize that a definitive "diet executioner" is your very own absence of poise and core interest.

During weight loss, you can covertly be the cause of all your problems.

If you've taken a stab at losing weight or a weight loss program previously, and have observed it be a difficult task where losing a couple of pounds to gain it all over again increasingly, then it is time that you think about what psychological cycle you go through and break out of it so you will reach your goal.

THE PSYCHOLOGICAL CYCLE OF WEIGHT GAIN

In this present reality where dainty is in, it's not surprising for people who are overweight to worry about the concern of lower confidence. Add to that the social shame or partiality that obese individuals experience and a psychological cycle for weight gain can be set moving or undesirable eating issue (bulimia, anorexia) can create.

People, overweight just as slight, regularly eat because of stress, sadness, forlornness, and tension. This pressure incited or enthusiastic eating can prompt weight gain, which thus inspires lower confidence, grief, and nervousness, which prompts more pressure-based overeating and extra weight gain. It's anything but difficult to perceive how one can wind up caught in a risky descending winding and endless loop.

Exacerbating the issue is the way that individuals who are overweight have less energy, and along these lines think that its harder to be dynamic, so the danger of gaining weight again increases. A cycle of idleness and further weight gain can build-up: the less dynamic individual gains weight thus turns out to be less dynamic, in this manner gaining more weight, etc. Likewise, life stresses, which are ordinarily mitigated through exercise, begin working up, which triggers more pressure-based eating.

Individuals who attempt to lose weight and come up short may feel discouraged, disappointed, and even liable or embarrassed and may depend on solace nourishments as an approach to feel better. The equivalent is valid for the individuals who prevail with regards to losing weight, to gain it back. Uneasiness, misery, and blame can deliver a feeling of sadness that upsets efforts to lose weight.

This is why jumping on the correct weight loss program is CRUCIAL for effective weight loss. Regardless of whether it's a weight loss diet that you've forced on yourself or a program intended for your body, pursue the following seven stages to break the psychological cycle of weight loss.

SEVEN STEPS TO BREAKING THE CYCLE

1. Stop Diet Deprivation. Diets and weight loss programs that put severe limitations on what you can eat often stimulate voraciously consuming food. While you may wait for some time, one day you'll choose to deny yourself isn't justified, despite any potential benefits, or you can't tolerate it any longer, and you dive into the more relaxed, cooler or nibble bureau furiously. Permit yourself little guilty pleasures that are fulfilling and will enable you to maintain a strategic distance from unsafe binging.

2. Plan Ahead. Imagine a scenario where you should slip. The ideal approach to abstain from slipping is through pre-planning. In this way, if you're set for a backyard grill or family assembling choose early what your plan is. Eat something substantial and rounding before you go out and after that permit yourself a couple of rare treats at the gathering, however, exercise a bit control. If you realize that Aunt Mary is making your preferred pastry, plan on having a little cut, and relish it. Dealing with your weight and getting a charge out of life ought to go connected at the hip.

3. Set Realistic Weight Loss Goals. To stay away from the dissatisfaction of falling flat, don't overemphasize yourself with ridiculous weight loss goals. You gained weight gradually after some time, and it will require some investment to lose that weight slowly. Slow, however, sure is the best approach.

4. Pick Healthy Outlets for Emotions. Rather than opening the fridge when you're upset, what about calling a companion, or go for a stroll.

Find something that makes you feel more settled or more joyful - something other than sustenance or liquor. Do yoga, move around your front room, ruminate, or go out bowling with a companion.

5. Quit Harboring Hurts. Work through issues that are upsetting you. Converse with a specialist or even a companion. Try not to give harms, a chance to even old injuries or examples that venture back into your adolescence, influence you and your association with sustenance.

6. Keep in mind Why You're Dieting. It stops and recollects why you're dieting in any case. Is it to have more energy, look and feel better, ease medical issues, or improve your confidence? Remembering the goal is essential to your weight loss achievement.

7. Utilize Your Mind to Break the Cycle. The truth of the matter is you can do it. It's all in your mind - the ability to lose the weight rests with you. Trust you can succeed, and you will achieve. If you need to put a conclusion to the psychological cycle of weight gain, begin by transforming the majority of your negative self-talk into positive affirmations. That is the ideal approach to break the cycle.

Rather than saying: "See that fat midsection. It just won't leave." Think positive: "Truly, my gut is fat now. However, it won't always be. I plan to be fit, not fat. I'm making a beeline for the rec centre after work today."

Remember your goal consistently. Record your positive affirmations and put up visual reminders of what you need to achieve - that dress you need to purchase, that ocean side hotel you're aching to visit this year, or even an image of the cheerful individual you need to be again. It's everything inside reach if you set your mind to it, keep dynamic, exercise, and plan substantial menus that you appreciate.

Utilize these seven stages to make a psychological turnaround and move pass the psychological hindrances that are keeping you down. If you do, you'll have the ability to accomplish lasting weight loss - something that will change your future and your life.

Chapter 27
Goal Setting

For many bariatric patients, goals are not a foreign concept. You've likely worked on your weight loss goals long before you ever thought about surgery as an option.

You likely know what your goals are. Yet, you are probably cynical, since up until now, it's been hard to reach them. Following bariatric surgery, it gets more comfortable because you see the amazing progress and you see it quickly. There are stalls in weight which can freak people out.

"Am I stuck? Will I continue to lose? Is this a plateau? How long will I be here (at this weight)?"

The panic sets in.

First, calm down. If you are doing what needs to be done, your weight will continue to drop. As you lose weight, your body is adjusting to a sharp decrease in food intake. You may want to discuss with your surgical team (bariatrician, dietician, etc.) regarding how many calories you are getting and whether you need to decrease or increase your caloric intake.

You may be shocked at this, but sometimes the reason people are not losing weight is that they are simply not eating enough and the body has engaged in starvation mode, so it is hanging on to every morsel in your body. Other times, you may need to reduce your calories to continue to experience weight loss. This is a very personal issue, and stalls do happen.

We all experience them. Some people experience stalls that last two weeks and some people experience stalls that last six weeks. This is when it's important to reach out to your physician or dietitian to evaluate what you may or may not be doing to help you drop. This is why awareness is essential. If you are eating off-plan and not aware, you're returning to autopilot behavior that may be causing you to gain the weight.

Another study found that when people were engaged in self-monitoring, they did a better job of losing weight and keeping the weight off (Odom et al., 2009). Self-monitoring consists of keeping a food journal, tracking exercise and other progress, as well as tracking water intake, supplements, and emotions.

It's a good idea to grab a food journal to track you're eating, on a day-to-day basis, so you are practicing the awareness of what you are eating. This helps you consciously process what you are about to put into your mouth or reflect on what you already ate on any given day. It's been shown that when you are more conscious of your choices, you make better ones.

It is important to be realistic about your goals, and it's essential that you discuss this with your surgeon as well. I also need to note here; for some individuals, the BMI chart can be deceiving.

This does not mean you get a free pass to bypass the BMI chart. However, it's important to see where you fall and whether it's a factor in your actual body fat percentage overall. As someone who is 5'11" tall, I know I'm never going to be 160lbs, and that is precisely what the chart shows I should be. I'm not saying that you should hide your head in the sand, or state you're 'big-boned' if you're not.

The goal is for you to lose weight and to be healthy for your body's height. It's all about proportion. The goal here is NOT to get you down to a specific weight per se, but to get you to a weight that YOU are comfortable at, and at a weight and size in which you feel good living in your body. You, feeling comfortable in your own body, makes all the difference.

Let's look at your personal goals for short-term and long-term, to help you gain an idea of where you want to be.

~ What are the realistic goals for your weight and height?

~ How much do you expect to lose overall?

~ What is your HEIGHT?

~ What was your HIGHEST weight?

~ What was your Surgery Weight?

~ What is your Current Weight?

~ What is your ideal ending Goal Weight?

~ What are your post-surgery (pounds lost) goals for:

Month 1:

What size do you want to be in?

How do you want to feel?

Month 3:

What size do you want to be in?

How do you want to feel?

Month 6:

What size do you want to be in?

How do you want to feel?

Month 9:

What size do you want to be in?

How do you want to feel?

Month 12:

What size do you want to be in?

How do you want to feel?

Month 18:

What size do you want to be in?

How do you want to feel?

Month 24:

What size do you want to be in?

How do you want to feel?

Month 30:

What size do you want to be in?

How do you want to feel?

Month 36:

What size do you want to be in?

How do you want to feel?

If you don't know what you want, how will you go after it?

Clarity is so important. Knowing what you want is step one. If you do not yet know what you will do once you lose the weight, start thinking about it now.

The plan is to lose weight and to do all the things you have not had the opportunity to do as an obese individual. There's so much more life for you to live and many things that I know you want to do.

~ Do you have a desire to travel to Europe and walk through the ancient streets of Rome?

~ Do you want to walk/run a 5k?

~ Do you want to chase after your grandchildren and be able to pick them up at a moment's notice?

~ Or would you like to feel comfortable making love to your husband/wife?

~ What is it that means the most to you?

~ What are those things that you're excited to do now that you're losing the weight?

List them out.

Chapter 28

The Rapid Weight Loss: Good or Bad?

No nourishment is taboo when you pursue this arrangement, which doesn't make you purchase any prepackaged suppers.

Rapid Weight Loss appoints different nourishments Point esteem. Nutritious nourishments that top you off have less focuses than garbage with void calories. The eating plan factors sugar, fat, and protein into its focuses counts to direct you toward natural products, veggies, and lean protein, and away from stuff that is high in sugar and immersed fat.

You'll have a Point focus on that is set up dependent on your body and objectives. For whatever length of time that you remain inside your everyday target, you can spend those Points anyway you'd like, even on liquor or treat, or spare them to utilize one more day.

However, more beneficial, lower-calorie nourishments cost less focuses. Furthermore, a few things presently have 0 points.

Level of Effort: Medium

Rapid Weight Loss is intended to make it simpler to change your propensities long haul, and it's adaptable enough that you ought to have the option to adjust it to your life. You'll improve your eating and lifestyle designs - a considerable lot of which you may have had for quite a long time - and you'll make new ones.

How much exertion it takes relies upon the amount you'll need to change your propensities.

Cooking and shopping: Expect to figure out how to shop, cook solid nourishments, and eat out in manners that help your weight-loss objective without holding back on taste or expecting to purchase strange nourishments.

Bundled nourishments or dinners: Not required.

In-person gatherings: Optional.

Exercise: You'll get a customized action objective and access to the program's application that tracks Points. You get acknowledgment for the entirety of your action.

Does It Allow for Dietary Restrictions or Preferences?

Because you pick how you spend your Points, you can at present do Rapid Weight Loss if you're a veggie-lover, vegetarian, have different inclinations, or if you have to confine salt or fat.

What Else You Should Know

Cost: Rapid Weight Loss offers three plans: Online just, online with gatherings, or online with one-on-one training through telephone calls and messages. Check the Rapid Weight Loss site for the evaluating for the online-just and online-with gatherings alternatives (you'll have to enter your ZIP code).

Costs and offers may differ.

Backing: Besides the discretionary in-person gatherings (presently called health workshops) and individual instructing, Rapid Weight Loss Program has an application, online network, a magazine, and a site with plans, tips, examples of overcoming adversity, and that's only the tip of the iceberg.

Does It Work?

Rapid Weight Loss is one of the well-looked into weight loss programs accessible. What's more, indeed, it works.

Numerous studies have demonstrated that the arrangement can assist you with getting more fit and keep it off.

For example, an investigation from The American Journal of Medicine demonstrated that individuals making Rapid Weight Loss lost more weight than those attempting to drop beats without anyone else.

Rapid Weight Loss positioned first both for "Best Weight Loss Diet" and for "Best Commercial Diet Plan" in the 2018 rankings from U.S. News and World Report.

Generally speaking, it's a great, simple to-pursue program.

Is It Good for Certain Conditions?

Rapid Weight Loss is useful for anybody. In any case, its attention on nutritious, low-calorie nourishments makes it extraordinary for individuals with hypertension, elevated cholesterol, diabetes, and even coronary illness.

If you pick any premade dinners, check the names, as some might be high in sodium.

Please work with your primary care physician so they can check your advancement, as well. This is particularly significant for individuals with diabetes, as you may need to alter your medication as you get in shape.

If the idea of gauging your nourishment or checking calories make your head turn, this is a perfect program because it takes every necessary step for you. The online instrument allocates a specific number an incentive to every nourishment, even eatery nourishments, to make it simple to remain on track.

If you don't have the foggiest idea about your way around the kitchen, the premade dinners and bites make it simple. They're a speedy and simple approach to control partition sizes and calories.

You don't need to drop any nourishment from your eating routine, yet you should constrain divide sizes to curtail calories.

The accentuation on foods grown from the ground implies the eating routine is high in fiber, which helps keep you full. Also, the program is easy to pursue, making it simpler to adhere to. You can likewise discover Rapid Weight Loss Program premade dinners at your neighborhood market.

A major favorable position of Rapid Weight Loss is their site. They offer exhaustive data on abstaining from excessive food intake, exercise, cooking, and wellness tips, just as online care groups.

Beset up to go through some cash to get the full advantages of the vigorous program. It tends to be somewhat expensive, yet it's well justified, despite all the trouble to harvest the wellbeing advantages of getting more fit and keeping it off.

Part Benefits

Dieters who join Rapid weight loss are known as "individuals."

Individuals can browse a few projects with differing levels of help.

An essential online program incorporates every minute of every day online visit support, just as applications and different instruments. Individuals can pay more for face to face bunch gatherings or one-on-one help from a Rapid weight loss individual mentor.

Individuals additionally get access to an online database of thousands of nourishments and plans, notwithstanding the following application for logging Points.

Also, Rapid weight loss supports physical action by relegating a wellness objective utilizing Points.

Every action can be signed into the Rapid weight loss application until the client arrives at their week after week FitPoint objective.

Exercises like moving, strolling and cleaning would all be able to be tallied towards your Point objective.

Rapid weight loss additionally gives wellness recordings and exercise schedules for their individuals.

Alongside diet and exercise directing, Rapid weight loss sells bundled nourishment like solidified suppers, cereal, chocolates and low-calorie dessert.

Outline

Rapid weight loss doles out guide esteems toward nourishments. Individuals must remain under their assigned day by day nourishment and drink focuses to meet their weight-misfortune objectives.

Would it be able to Help You Lose Weight?

Rapid weight loss utilizes a science-based way to deal with weight misfortune, accentuating the significance of part control, nourishment decisions and moderate, predictable weight misfortune.

Dissimilar to numerous craze diets that guarantee unreasonable outcomes over brief timeframes, Rapid weight loss discloses to individuals that they ought to hope to lose .5 to 2 pounds (.23 to .9 kg) every week.

The program features lifestyle modification and advice individuals on the best way to settle on better choices by utilizing the Points framework, which organizes sound nourishments.

Numerous studies have demonstrated that Rapid weight loss can help with weight misfortune.

Rapid weight loss gives a whole page of their site to scientific examinations supporting their program.

One study found that overweight individuals who were advised to get more fit by their PCPs lost twice as a lot of weight on the Rapid weight loss program than the individuals who got standard weight misfortune directing from essential care proficient.

Even though this investigation was subsidized by Rapid weight loss, information gathering and examination were facilitated by a free research group.

Besides, an audit of 39 controlled examinations found that members following the Rapid weight loss program lost 2.6% more weight than members who got different sorts of guiding.

Another controlled investigation in more than 1,200 hefty grown-ups found that members who pursued the Rapid weight loss program for one year lost significantly more weight than the individuals who got self-improvement materials or brief weight-misfortune counsel.

Besides, members following Rapid weight loss for one year were increasingly fruitful at keeping up their weight misfortune for more than two years, contrasted with different gatherings.

Rapid weight loss is one of only a handful scarcely any weight-misfortune programs with demonstrated outcomes from randomized controlled preliminaries, which are considered the "best quality level" of therapeutic research.

Chapter 29
Keeping Up with Nutrition

Eating Healthy Vs. Achieving Your Goal Physique

With the idea of attaining a fantastic body, folks instantly consider eating healthy. Nevertheless, eating healthful foods does not automatically mean that you're achieving your target body. While obtaining your very best body does not exactly mean that you're eating healthy. To eat healthily means typically you give your body with sufficient nutrients to operate effectively. Your body needs a particular number of micronutrients (vitamins and minerals) and macronutrients (carbohydrates, proteins, and carbohydrates) to work in its very best ability. You must satisfy your body's nutrient requirements to keep decent health. Reaching a fantastic body usually involves losing weight or gaining muscle. To be able to lose excess weight, a person must maintain a calorie deficit wherever your body burns off more calories than the number of calories you eat and drink. Gaining weight requires you to do the contrary, at which in a calorie excess you have more calories than the amount the body burns off calories off.

Though eating healthful foods has unlimited benefits, It's just as important to satisfy the necessity of attaining your exercise goal. By way of example, if your objective is to burn fat and you also eat 10,000 calories worth of veggies every day, you are eating healthy but are consuming a lot of calories to achieve your objective. Because of this, it's best to consume towards your target body when keeping excellent health.

What's a Calorie?

You hear about calories all of the time, but what does it mean? A calorie is a device that measures energy. The food that you eat is not measured in size or weight, but by how much energy it's. If you hear something that includes 100 calories, it is a method of describing just how much energy your body might gain from drinking or eating it. As the quantity of gas pumped into a vehicle is measured in gallons, different food, or beverages you eat is measured in calories. The body breaks down food in an exceptional manner, so the number of calories is a means of understanding how much energy your system will get from whatever you eat or drink. 'Calorie' is only a specialized phrase for 'energy'.

Are Calories Bad For You?

Calories aren't bad for you because the body needs them to get energy. Nevertheless, eating a lot of calories and not burning off enough of these off through physical activity may cause weight gain with time. Consuming too small calories over time won't enable your body to work properly and may harm your wellbeing. Foods like lettuce contain hardly any calories (1 cup of shredded lettuce has less than ten calories). In contrast, foods such as peanuts have plenty of calories (1/2 cup of peanuts contains 427 calories daily). Understanding how many calories your body requires each day can allow you to select which foods are right for you.

How Does Your Body Use Calories?

Your body requires calories simply to remain alive and function properly. This energy is utilized for basic functions like maintaining your heart beating and lung breathing. Calories are crucial for several fundamental and intricate functions such as the regulation of body temperature as well as also the functioning of each cell in the human entire body. The more activity you do will be that the more calories you burn off. Your body also requires calories to grow and grow. You burn calories before considering it as during the digestion of food, recovery of muscles after exercise, as well as while you are sleeping.

How Many Calories Do You Want?

Folks differ in size and have different metabolisms; therefore, the number of calories an individual should eat will change based upon many things. These factors include an individual's height, age, weight, and daily activity level. The larger an individual is, the more calories a person could want, vice versa. Although two individuals can have exactly the identical body dimensions, the number of calories that they want can differ due to the way their body adjusts exactly what they eat. Calorie calculators are available on the internet, which may be employed to ascertain the number of calories your body requires depends on the vital facets. If you consume many calories than your body wants, then the additional calories are converted to fat. If you consume fewer calories than you require, then your system uses your stored body fat as the energy it needs to function. Knowing the number of calories you want can allow you to control your weight.

Macro Basics

Macronutrients or macros are carbs, fats, and protein. Together with the expression "macro," meaning quite big, these three nutrients are responsible for supplying calories (the only other material that supplies calories is alcohol, however, isn't a macronutrient because we don't want it for survival). Whatever that you eat is broken down into those three macronutrients. Your body doesn't recognize the food that you consume as "poultry, sausage, rice, etc." Rather, your entire body sees anything you eat as a carbohydrate, fat, or protein. This is why you find these macronutrients written in bold letters to the nutrition label of any food or beverage product.

What's a Carb?

Carbohydrate is the body's main source of energy. There are two kinds of carbohydrates, complex and simple. A very simple carbohydrate supplies your body with rapid energy but does not last long. An intricate carbohydrate takes more time to break down on your body; nevertheless, it is a long-lasting supply of energy. Neither simple nor complex carbohydrate is bad for you. They could both be utilized to your benefit throughout the day. Upon waking in the morning, you likely have not had anything to eat for the past couple of hours you have been asleep. Therefore it is sometimes a fantastic idea to eat simple carbohydrates for instant energy. If you intend on being from home for a couple of hours, complex carbohydrates are a great selection for its long-term steady energy. So integrating both kinds of carbohydrates in your diet may permit you better to manage your levels of energy throughout the day.

Examples of complex carbohydrates include whole grains like whole Wheat bread, oatmeal, and brown rice alongside other foods like sweet potato and beans. Simple carbs include foods like fruits, white bread, white rice, white potatoes, veggies, juice, pop tarts, etc. Sugar is a simple carbohydrate that comes in various forms like sugar, fructose, lactose, sucrose, etc. Though both intricate and straightforward carbohydrates are broken down to glucose within the body, absorption and digestion are the principal differences between both different types.

What Is Protein?

Protein helps build and repair tissue when playing a role in various cell functions within the body. It's a significant element for growing nails, hair, muscle, and different areas of the human body. Amino acids are building blocks of protein. An entire protein includes all 20 amino acids, even while the lack of one or more amino acids is known as an incomplete protein. Complete proteins are primarily found in meats like poultry, beef, beef, and fish in addition to legumes, milk, and whey protein. Foods like grains, seeds, nuts, or beans are considered incomplete proteins. It's encouraged to eat at least 0.8 - 1.2 g of protein per 1 pound of your body weight for optimum muscle development. With several unique forms of protein in the marketplace which range from the origin, absorption rate, and procedure of filtration, any comprehensive protein is helpful for the growth and repair of muscle. Poultry, fish, milk, legume, soy, whey, and other resources of proteins have their differences, but any comprehensive protein is of fantastic advantage for repairing and building muscle. The crucial thing is to find sufficient protein to satisfy your body's need for optimum growth.

What Is Fat?

Fat controls hormones, aides from the transportation of cells, and makes it feasible for different nutrients to finish tasks within the body. Fat can also be your body's secondary source of vitality. When your body doesn't have sufficient carbohydrates easily available, it uses fat as an alternative source of gas. As a result, the notion of burning fat is to limit the quantity of primary energy (carbohydrates) so the body can utilize its secondary resource of energy (body fat). Various kinds of fats contain saturated fat, polyunsaturated, monounsaturated, and trans-fat. It's encouraged to steer clear of trans-fat because of its health advantages. While every kind of fat has its advantages and disadvantages, it's helpful to look closely at the whole amount of fat in a single product.

Foods that have a high number of fat include peanut butter, oils, avocado, and nuts. Consuming low levels of fat over the years may lead to hormone levels to become erratic, which makes it important to have enough even while attempting to burn off fat. The quantity of fat required daily could vary anywhere from 15 percent to over 40 percent of total calories based on the person and fitness target.

Quality of Weight Loss or Weight Gain

If you're in a calorie deficit where your body burns off more calories than you eat, then you are going to eliminate weight. This doesn't automatically make sure that the entire weight you lose is only going to come from fat. Your body is composed of lean mass, fat, and fat. This implies any weight that's lost or obtained may come from any one of those three. When shedding fat, you risk losing weight, and if gaining weight, you risk placing on excess fat. Not monitoring macros puts you at a greater risk for muscle loss and fat gain since you would not understand how many calories you're becoming. Consuming the ideal amount of protein, fat, and carbohydrates helps to make sure you keep muscle while shedding weight, and restrict the rise of body fat while incorporating muscle.

More Energy, Better Mood

Carbohydrates are the body's most important source of energy, therefore getting too little carbohydrates over time may leave you feeling exhausted and contribute to inadequate workout functionality. By properly setting up your macros, you optimize the number of carbohydrates you can consume while burning off fat. If you may eat more food while losing weight, then why not make the most of fat is in charge of controlling your hormones, therefore not having sufficient can lead to an imbalance that could result in mood swings and other undesirable symptoms. It's normal to drop short of your everyday fat requirements by merely eating "clean" foods that typically include little to no fat. Consuming low fat and carbohydrates over time may allow you to feel exceptionally miserable. To believe losing weight is a struggle, why make it tougher on yourself to accomplish your objective.

Chapter 30
The Practice of BioBalancing

This is your life. This moment. Here and now. The place you want to be is here and now. The person you want to be is right here, right now. The best that life has to offer isn't somewhere else. Life can only be lived right where you are, at this moment. But the question is… is your mind present here and now?

The reason I ask is that the act of BioBalancing is a very mindful skill. BioBalancing is like an anchor into the present moment. Each time you check-in with yourself, you are mindful. Each time you cater to your needs, you are displaying the mindful traits of compassion and love. This can have a powerfully positive knock-on effect for the rest of your life.

This is how this works:

The more you practice BioBalancing, the more clarity and understanding you'll have of your internal emotional landscape. It motivates and drives you to your desire. Your true needs and wants become apparent. Your core values become more defined. You won't get some glaring flashing sign or signal, it's much subtler than that, just a general feeling of when something is "right" and when something is "wrong" for you—a sort of deep sense of wisdom. You'll know, deep in your soul. Once you get a clearer indication of what makes you happy, you can start to align your life accordingly to achieve more of it.

I believe this is the secret key to true happiness. It's not about getting more stuff, a bigger house or a fancier car. It's about you tapping into the real you and discovering what makes you truly fulfilled and happy. It's what we all want deep down. To live a happy life. To experience that true happiness that sinks deep into your bones and effects everything you do.

To do this, follow the 3 BioBalance principles:

1. Nourish: Ensure you are addressing your core needs.

2. Observe: Observe your emotional landscape within your body and discover what's important to you.

3. Rebalance: Figure out what you need to do to achieve more of what you want at a deeper level.

You know, recently I've become passionate about taking my family out for walks. I love staring at the scenery, watching the grass, feeling the wind and just being amazed. That abundance, that feeling of life, it's blissful. This is something I have discovered I enjoy from tapping into my body sense.

My life has changed in so many positive ways since I started listening to my internal guidance system. That's not to say my life is all sunshine and roses, it still certainly has its fair share of challenges, but when you're connected to the true you, when you're feeling balanced and when you nourish your core needs, life flows a lot smoother. A profound shift occurs in how you feel, in how you interact with others, in your relationships, your sense of self, your productivity. Everything.

Balance NOT perfection

What you need to keep in mind is that we're striving for a more balanced life, not a perfect life (perfection doesn't exist, and it's a sure-fire path to misery). The keyword is "striving". We are never, ever, truly perfectly balanced. Like a tree blowing in the wind, we need to allow ourselves to sway from side to side when the wind blows. Our life needs to be flexible, and we need to be open to and accepting of whatever crops up in the present moment. Life can throw us a curveball at any moment, and we need to be ready to accept that. The key is to have an attitude of always striving for balance while becoming more accepting of unexpected changes and outcomes (this includes setbacks and relapses!).

So learn to trust your inner wisdom, your instincts, and your body awareness. If it feels right for you, it is right for you. If it doesn't feel right, then change it. All the wisdom and knowledge you need is already there, inside you.

The great thing about BioBalancing is that it is a skill. It's something you can get better throughout your life. It is a process of self-discovery in the truest sense. It's a wonderful journey of self-exploration, and it helps to strengthen, nurture and enhance the most important relationship in your life: The one you have with yourself.

Chapter 31
The Conditions of Manifesting

The 8 Conditions of Manifesting

How to begin the process of manifesting.

Now, how to will be given.

Step 1:

You've discovered this fantastic idea called the Law of Attraction which promises "all of your dreams can become a reality. "Everything is getting more exciting. You perform a basic Google search for "how to manifest" or some similar search term. What do you find? Approximately 200 million results! The most common formula presented is one coined from popular books and the movie, The Secret, all which suggest there are three simple steps to the Law of Attraction.

Countless listings suggest you can use "7 steps to manifest anything you want"—or maybe 5 or 4. Perhaps, you'll see "how to manifest overnight" or "manifest instantly." The options go on…and on. The list of formulas, processes, systems, step-by-step strategies is endless. Each promotes a similar thinking strategy, "follow these steps in this particular order, and all your dreams will come true."

Step 2:

Figure out which one of these approaches makes the most sense for you and start following each step.

Step 3:

After anywhere from 1-to-7 days, to even God forbid, 30 days or more trying to manifest what you want, you find yourself in a dilemma. There you sit, still trying to manifest what you want. Now you're thinking, "Yup, just like I thought all along, the Law of Attraction doesn't work!" Sound familiar?

Yet, somewhere deep inside you, you still long to believe. This stuff is out there for a reason so being resilient; you get up, dust yourself off, and try again—even harder this time. And again, you fail to get the results you want! Now you have double the data and double the discouragement.

What happened?

Here's the deal. While each of these approaches has some truth to them, the strategy is somewhat flawed, when presented as a linear, step-by-step process.

The Law of Attraction is not a step-by-step, one-size-fits-all process, and it's not linear.

A linear process is something that progresses directly from one stage to another with a starting point and an ending point.

LOA is most often described as a process because it's easier to explain and market the concept that way.

I'm willing to risk going against all those other processes to share the truth from my experience. The Law of Attraction is a bit messier than what's popularly suggested. If you want to make it work, I suggest following good old Einstein's wise words, "If you want different results, you have to try different approaches."

My experiences show that manifesting is best described in non-linear terms. I say it does not progress or advance like phases, going in some logical sequence. Rather, "Law of Attraction is when the manifesting conditions and personal qualities are developed and come into alignment simultaneously."

Each condition plays an important role in manifesting. And they do not always happen in the order in which they will appear in this text. These conditions can all be in play at once.

Law of Attraction is about being in alignment with all eight of the manifesting conditions, simultaneously.

The "formula," if you will, is to work through each of the conditions for manifesting only. By doing this, you will gain an understanding of what it means to be in alignment with that condition. Be sure to do the exercise assignments to support your endeavor further.

Think of it a little like juggling eight balls at a time. Start by getting good at juggling the one ball. Then add a second, and a third. With practice, soon, you will learn to juggle all eight balls at once. This is when you are in alignment with your manifestation.

The time it takes is the time it takes. Seriously! You can be in alignment with all eight conditions within a matter of a second, or it can take 20 years. It all depends on how quickly or slowly you get into alignment with each condition. But the moment you are in alignment, a manifestation is instant.

The Manifesting Conditions:

Condition #1 Desire

Defined: A strong feeling of wanting to have something or wishing for something to happen.

Condition #2 Thought

Defined: An idea or opinion produced by thinking or occurring suddenly in the mind.

Condition #3 Imagination

Defined: The formation of a mental image of something. Form a mental picture of; imagine.

Condition #4 Belief/Expectancy

Defined: Accept as real; feel sure of the truth of.

Condition #5 Feeling/Vibration

Defined: An emotional state or reaction.

Condition #6 Creative Attraction

Defined: The action or power of drawing forth a response: an attractive quality.

Condition #7 Inspired Action

Defined: The process of doing something, arising from creative impulse, to achieve something extraordinary.

Condition #8 Manifestation

Defined: To make evident or certain by showing or displaying.

Chapter 32
Guide to Helping Move Forward

Now that you have learned all of the components to changing your life for the better when it comes to emotional eating, I am going to leave you with some tips to make sure that you can stay on track and achieve your goals. One of the keys to this that I want to begin with is going into it intending to combine everything you have learned and want to accomplish into one new lifestyle for yourself. This will include your new meal plans, your new snack options, and choices, your continued work on your relationship with food and with yourself, as well as regular exercise. As you begin, it will be difficult, but ease your way into it. And once these all become habits, you won't even notice that you are doing them anymore, and they will become second nature. Anything can become a habit if we practice it for long enough, and these lifestyle changes are no different.

What to Do When It Becomes Difficult

It is inevitable when trying to accomplish something as big as making a change to something that is ingrained in your life- like eating, that it will become difficult at some points along the way. This part will look at what we can do when it becomes painful.

The first thing that you should do is expect it to become difficult at some point. Going into this journey, hoping that it will be a breeze, will only leave you feeling like you have done something wrong when a hard day or a tough week surprises you if you go into this if the mindset that it will become difficult at least a few times, will prevent this from surprising you when it happens and will allow you to appropriately deal with it instead of wondering what you did you cause it.

When it becomes difficult, and you don't know what to eat, you are in a rush, and you have no groceries left, the first thing you want to do is take a deep breath. Then, remind yourself why you started in the very first place. Think back on your old ways and how they made you feel. Think of where you are now and praise yourself for what you have accomplished so far- no matter how small. Then, go to the fridge and eat one of the lunches you had intended to take for work tomorrow. By tomorrow, you will likely be having a better day and will have regrouped with your old willpower restored, which will allow you to make a right and healthy decision for your lunch.

Don't get discouraged when something arises that challenges you on your journey. Take it as it comes and tell yourself that this is just what happens in life. Nothing comes without challenges. If something comes up that causes you to slip up and eat something that you would otherwise have chosen not to, don't beat yourself up; just continue with your plan and continue as you would have at the next meal.

Motivation Tips

When you lack motivation, it will help to write about this in your workbook. Sometimes when things become a habit, we forget that they didn't use to be. Think about some of the things that are habits of yours now that were not habits of yours a year ago. This will remind you of what you can accomplish.

Reach out to someone who is supporting you that can provide you with some words of encouragement. This could be anyone who you trust and who you know has your best interests at heart. They will be able to give you some words to motivate you and keep you on track.

Look to support centers online for people recovering from emotional eating or other food-related issues. This can help you to feel that you are not alone and that many other people are facing similar challenges. This will motivate you to keep pushing.

How to Work on Willpower

Willpower is hard to pinpoint, but that is somewhere within all of us. We have to find it somewhere within, and it is there! Think of someone or some people who you think to demonstrate great willpower. Ask yourself what about them shows this. Ask yourself how you think they do this (don't reply with "they just have it"). Ask yourself what other qualities they possess that you admire. Ask yourself if you can pull those same qualities from within yourself. Thinking in this way and trying to emulate a person you admire and respect will help you to know precisely how willpower looks to you and how willpower displays itself in a person. Having something more concrete to work towards or to reference will help you to find the willpower that is within you.

How to Stick to the Diet

The key to sticking to the diet is one word: preparation. Being prepared for anything will ensure that you won't be able to give yourself any excuse to fall off of the diet. For example, doing all of the following:

· Meal prep your lunches.

· Find a place to buy a healthy lunch near your work or school, just in case you forget your lunch one day.

· Prepare a menu for your dinners for the week each weekend.

· Don't buy the snacks that you would usually crave at the grocery store.

· Grocery shop with a specific list and when you are not hungry.

· If you are going out socially, pre-plan what you will order and the number and type of drinks you will have. Then stick to this.

Doing all of the above things will make it almost impossible to not stick to the diet. Because everything will be prepared for you already, all you have to do is move the fork to your mouth at every meal, and the diet is stuck to!

How to Reward Yourself as You Hit Milestones

Rewarding yourself is vital as you make your way through this challenging journey. When you hit milestones like one month on the diet or one month without giving in to a craving, then you will keep yourself motivated because you will be working toward your next milestone and, therefore, your next reward each day. Leave enough space between rewards; otherwise, they won't feel as unique. Reward yourself once per month at first and then once every few months as you get more used to everything. You can reward yourself by allowing yourself to buy a medium popcorn at the movie theatre after you have exercised three times a week for a month, for example.

Plan your rewards and write them down on a calendar so that if you are feeling a lack of motivation, you will be able to look at the visual and see how close you are to achieving that goal and that reward. We as creatures love to be rewarded and love to accomplish goals and so giving yourself these options will help you to achieve them.

Chapter 33
The Intermittent Fasting

Especially intermittent fasting isn't hunger. Needing is a modified restriction to eat by power by outside forces; it occurs amid war and starvation when there isn't adequate sustenance. Fasting, on the other hand, is settled, wise and controlled. Sustenance is instantly open, anyway, we choose not to eat it for huge reasons, a success for a couple of reasons.

Fasting is as old as humankind, obviously more settled than the various types of weight control plans. Obsolete urban foundations, for instance, the Greeks, found that there was something significant for infrequent fasting. They are conventionally known as spillage, cleansing, filtration or detoxification. Every culture and religion on earth applies for two or more fasting shows.

Before the closeness of agriculture, people never ate up three suppers dependably, paying little heed to whether they ate at the centre. We ate well when we found sustenance that could be segregated for an impressive period of days. Starting now and into the foreseeable future, from development, three dinners day by day are emphatically not essential for endurance. Else, we should not be viewed as fit as creatures.

Quickly in the 21st century, the overall negligence of this out of date practice showed. The dispersion is deplorable for the movement! Sustenance boss requests us to eat a collection from dinners and snacks for a couple of days. Nutritionists alert that avoiding a single dinner will have basic flourishing results. Besides, these messages were so particularly entered in our psyches.

The circulation has no standard range. It will, in general, be produced from a couple of hours to a couple of days or even months. From time to time, fasting is a dietary structure wherein we move among fasting and a run of the mill eating schedule. Fasting, from under 4 pm to 8 pm, happens significantly more regularly than envisioned, even every day. An increasingly broadened fast, ordinarily 24 to 36 hours, is done 2 to multiple times every week. By chance, the overall made a walk by-step, all around requested around 12 hours among dinner and breakfast.

For quite a while, fasting has been a monster to a number of people. Is it troublesome? No, believe it or not, a couple of tests have shown that it has fantastic issue zones for prescriptions.

What happens when we eat consistently?

Before keeping an eye on the benefits of erratic fasting, it is perfect to understand why eating 5 to 6 dinners consistently or in a foreseen way (positive pivot fasting) can bring more toxicity than everything else.

When we eat, we eat a healthy target. The key hormone included is insulin (transmitted through the pancreas), which adds during dinner.

Sugar and protein increase insulin. Fat causes a slight change in insulin, but at this point and again it is eaten alone.

Insulin has two noteworthy obstacles:

• First and foremost, it empowers the body to start using most of its sustenance quickly. Starch rapidly changes over to glucose, growing glucose levels. Insulin guides glucose to the body's cells for accommodating use. Proteins are isolated in amino acids, and rich amino acids can be changed into glucose. Proteins don't grow glucose so much, yet they can manufacture insulin. Fats incidentally influence insulin.

• Secondly, insulin stores plenitude substances for later. Insulin changes over excess glucose into glycogen and stores it in the liver. In any case, the proportion of glycogen that can be managed is limited. Right when the camouflaged target disappears, the liver begins to change over glucose into fat. Fat is set up in the liver (richness) or in the muscle to fat proportions stores (never-ending save as ordinary or intestinal fat).

So when we eat and nibble for the day, we are constantly invigorated, and our insulin levels remain high. In the end, we could spend a not too bad bit of the day managing the nuts and bolts.

What happens when we speed?

The best approach to use and keep up the vital essential that develops when we eat goes the other way when we fast. Insulin levels decay, which makes the body start eating. Glycogen, glucose that the liver arrangements with, is first eaten up and used. Starting there, the body begins to disengage the muscles and fats in one of a kind way.

This way, the body on a very basic level exists in two conditions: an eating routine high in insulin and a fasting state low in insulin. We deal with the necessity for assistance or consume by far most of our jobs. In circumstances where diet and fasting are balanced, there is no weight gain. If we go through various days eating and profiting however much as could reasonably be expected from it, we are most likely going to consume extra time.

Unpredictable fasting versus consistent caloric control

The foreseen deficient control structure for calorie abatement is the most critical dietary recommendation for weight decrease and type 2 diabetes. For example, the American Diabetes Association recommends a deficiency of 500 to 750 kcal/day related to the activity of normal material science. Dietitians search for this procedure and propose eating someplace in the scope of 4 and 6 little meals every day.

Does the part control system work after some time? From time to time. A report by an assistant after a nine-year follow-up by the United Kingdom, of 176,495 gigantic individuals, exhibited that 3,528 had put on common body weight before starting the action. The mistake rate is 98%!

Wrong fasting is certainly not a relentless caloric control. The caloric restriction achieves a compensatory increase in the squeezing need and, what's all the more disturbing? A reduction in the metabolic rate in the body copies the experience of the hands! As we, for the most part, useless calories, it is continuously difficult to stay fit and essentially less recover weight ensuing to losing it. This sort of routine eating routine places the body in "hunger mode", and the treatment diminishes the extent essential.

A destroyed dispersion has none of these bothers.

Great remedial states of irregular fasting absorb weight increment, and muscle issues appear differently about fat.

Not the scarcest piece, a calorie decreasing eating routine, changed fasting grows absorption. That looks extraordinary from an endurance point of view. If we don't eat, the body uses the covered fundamental as fuel to stay alive and finds another dinner. The hormones empower the body to go from a wellspring of prerequisite for an eating routine to a solid or fat extent.

Focuses unmistakably show this wonder. For example, four days of uncommon fasting extended the basal metabolic rate by 12%. The degrees of the norepinephrine neural connection, which prepares the body for improvement, extended by 117%. Unsaturated fats in the stream structure outperformed 370% when the body changed from eating sustenance to losing fat.

In no condition is a strong eating routine to eat calories, broken fasting eats up muscles that feared a relative number of people. In 2010, experts investigated a lot of respondents, who experienced 70 days of fasting (one day of fasting and a related snappy). Its weight began at 52.0 kg and completed at 51.9 kg. In the end, there was no muscle adversity; they had lost 11.4% of their fat regardless and saw basic upgrades in LDL cholesterol levels and triglycerides.

During fasting, the body reliably moves the potentiating human hormone, which a tiny bit at a time extras muscles and slight bones. The mass is usually verified until the muscle/fat extent falls underneath 4%. Hence, it is unimaginable that a great number of people lose muscle when fasting.

Impels insulin impediment, type 2 diabetes and oily liver.

Type 2 diabetes is a sickness depicted by an unprecedented extent of sugar in the body, to the point that the body can never react to insulin and ingest more glucose in the blood (an insulin inhibitor), hence achieving a lot of glucose, bounty glucose when taken and managed.

To change this state, two things must happen:

• Stop setting more sugar in your body first.

• Consume the rest of the sugar.

The best diet to achieve this is an eating routine low in starch, free of protein and fat, furthermore called the ketogenic diet. (Remember that starch manufactures glucose, protein and less fat). That is the explanation, and a low carb diet will help reduce glucose weight. For specific people, this is adequate to change the control of insulin and type 2 diabetes. In all cases, in fabulously dishonorable cases, the eating routine itself isn't worthy.

Shouldn't I say something in regards to work out? Exercise will help with skeletal muscle glucose; anyway, there are very few tissues and organs left, including the oily liver. Without a doubt, the preparation is enormous. Any way to get glucose from the fruition of the organs, it is imperative to "fast" the cells quickly.

A wrecked creation can achieve this. That is the explanation people have called it, cleaning or detoxification. Generally, it will be an incredible ideal situation to discard a lot of surpluses. This is the snappiest strategy to reduce blood glucose, and insulin levels, in conclusion, put an end to the insulin deterrent, type 2 diabetes and oily liver.

Incidentally, taking insulin for sort two diabetes doesn't deal with the fundamental issue of excess sugar in the body. Security shows that insulin will expel glucose from your blood, empowering you to lower blood glucose, at any rate, where does the sugar go? The liver will change everything to fat, fat in the liver and fat in the stomach area.

[illegible]

[illegible]

Conclusion

Let's look back at our progress and then paying it forward to others. Ensure you revisit all the things you subscribed to while reading this book. Continue eating better all day. You'll feel better, look better, achieve your goals, and have a better quality of life. Assuming you've read and understood all the content in this book, chances are that you've realized your habits and applying core solutions to overcoming obstacles while holding yourself accountable, you have Paid attention to yourself, your purpose, unique talents, and dreams. By automating your food and water, cutting out unhealthy sugar, alcohol and white carbs, adding protein, Greek yogurt or other probiotics, produce and healthy fats.

Choose to continue with the same eating habit all your life. Focus on a healthy weight; stay with silence. Visualize your step and take steps that are going to get you to where you want to be. Destabilize procrastination, stress, comfort zone- you will go farther at a fast pace. Organize your kitchen and automate your food. Be a reader; Read positive affirmations aloud every day. Pursue your goals, including your fitness and health goals that will utilize your talents and passions and keep you on the healthy fit journey. Rest on weekends and follow the process again.

Focus on your activities, journalize your progress, thoughts, and move on. Record your success, nature; they will guide you in thinking and solving stress, among other problems. You will make not only an impact on yourself but also the people around you. Make use of productivity apps on the internet to guide you through.

While writing your journal, consider how you've grown physically, mentally, spiritually, and emotionally or socially. Think about how one area has positively affected other areas. If some things haven't worked out for you, spend some time forgiving other people, forgiving yourself so you can move on. Giving makes living worthwhile.

Albert Einstein believed that a life shared with others is worthy. We have people out there who need you, remember not to hoard your successes. Share your success. Share your new-found recipes, your attitude, and your habits. Share what you have learned with others. In all your undertakings, know that you can't change other people but yourself, therefore, be mindful. Reflect on your changes and Put yourself on the back today and every day. Be grateful and live your life as a champion.

Make it a reality on your mind the fact that the journey to a healthy life and weight loss is long and has many challenges. Pieces of Stuff we consider more important in life require our full cooperation towards them. Just because you are facing problems in your Wight loss journey, it does not mean that you should stop, instead show and prove the whole world how good your ability to handle constant challenges is — training your brain to know that eating healthy food together with functional exercises can work miracles. Make it your choice and not something you are forced to do by a third party. Always tell yourself that weight loss is a long process and not an event. Take every day of your days to celebrate your achievements because these achievements are what piles up to massive victory. Make a list of stuff you would like to change when you get healthy they may be Small size-clothes, being able to accumulate enough energy, participating in your most loved sports you have been admiring for a more extended period, feeling self-assured. Make these tips your number one source of empowerment; you will end up completing your 30 days even without noticing.

You have made it, or you are about to make it. The journey has been unbelievable. And by now, you must be having a story to tell. Concentrate on finishing strongly. Keep up the excellent eating design you have adopted. Remember, you are not working on temporary changes but long term goals. Therefore, lifestyle changes should not be stopped when the weight is lost. Remind yourself always of essential habits that are easier to follow daily. They include; trusting yourself and the process by acknowledging that the real change lies in your hands. Stop complacency, arise, and walk around for at least thirty minutes away. Your breakfast is the most important meal you deserve. Eat your breakfast like a queen. For each diet, you take, add a few proteins and natural fats. Let hunger not kill you, eat more, but just what is recommended, bring snacks and other meals 3- five times a day. Have more veggies and fruits like 5-6 rounds in 24 hours. Almost 90% of Americans do not receive enough vegetables and fruits to their satisfaction. Remember, Apple will not make you grow fat. Substitute salt. You will be shocked by the sweet taste of food once you stop consuming salt. Regain your original feeling you will differentiate natural flavorings from artificial flavors. Just brainstorm how those older adults managed to eat their food without salt or modern-day characters. Characters are not suitable for your health. Drink a lot of water in a day. Let water be your number one drink. Avoid soft drinks and other energy drinks, and they are slowly killing you. Drink a lot of water in the morning after getting out of your bed. Your body will be fresh from morning to evening. Have a journal, and be realistic with it. Take charge of what you write and be responsible.

CPSIA information can be obtained
at www.ICGtesting.com
Printed in the USA
LVHW011950241020
669606LV00012BA/424

9 781838 237172